THE PERRICONE PROMISE

Look Younger, Live Longer in
Three Easy Steps

NICHOLAS PERRICONE, M.D.

timewarner
books

A *Time Warner* Book

First published in the US by
Time Warner Book Group US, 2004
This edition published by
Time Warner Book Group UK, 2005

The program herein is not intended to replace the services of trained health professionals, or be a substitute for medical advice. You are advised to consult with your health care professional with regard to matters relating to your health, and in particular regarding matters that may require diagnosis or medical attention.

Several of the recipes in this book have been adapted with permission from *The Whole Food Bible: How to Select & Prepare Safe, Healthful Foods* by Chris Kilham, Healing Arts Press, Rochester, VT 05767
Copyright © 1991, 1997 by Chris Kilham www.InnerTraditions.com.

A CIP catalogue record for this book is available from the British Library.

ISBN 0 316 72996 5

Book design by L&G McRee
Printed and bound in Great Britain by
Clays Ltd, St Ives plc

Time Warner Books
An imprint of
Time Warner Book Group UK
Brettenham House
Lancaster Place
London WC2E 7EN

www.twbg.co.uk

To my children
Jeffrey, Nicholas, and Caitie

Acknowledgments

Anne Sellaro again deserves star billing in these acknowledgments. Anne's untiring enthusiasm, hard work, creativity, and vision as friend, agent, producer, and collaborator continue to help me share my message and mission with millions of people worldwide.

To Diana Baroni, my extraordinary editor at Warner Books, and the entire Warner team, including publicity expert Jennifer Romanello, the sales reps, and the marketing folks.

And to all of my friends and colleagues, including:

Eddie Magnotti

Tony Tiano, Lennlee Keep, Eli Brown, and the team at Santa Fe Productions

The Public Broadcasting Service (PBS-TV)

Desiree Gruber and the team at Full Picture

Richard Post

Our retail partners Neiman Marcus, Nordstrom, Sephora, Saks, Henri Bendel, and Clyde's on Madison

Tucker and Josh Greco, Dr. Dale Webb, Kevin Gors

Craig Weatherby

Steve Mirabella Sr.

The staff at N.V. Perricone, M.D., Ltd.

My parents

My brother and sisters, Jimmy, Laura, June, and Barbara

My children, Jeffrey, Nicholas, and Caitie

Beth and Ken Lazer and their children, Kyle, Jack, Dave, and Eric

Sharyn Kolberg

Contents

Introduction

Writing *The Perricone Promise* has been a great joy for me, because it has allowed me to introduce the latest breakthrough in fighting the cause of aging and age-related diseases: peptides and neuropeptides.

Whether your goal is to try to prevent serious diseases, such as cancer or heart disease, or simply to have wrinkle- or blemish-free skin, the three simple steps outlined in this book will provide both immediate and long-term age-defying benefits.

This might seem like a pretty lofty claim, but once you understand how it works, it will make perfect sense. My goal is not to introduce you to some wonder drug but rather to enable you to take control of your body and the rate at which it is aging—and actually help you put on the brakes.

In *The Perricone Promise,* I introduce powerful peptides and neuropeptides formulated into various products that have significant anti-inflammatory benefits at the cellular level. (Since inflammation occurs on a cellular level, our tools for fighting the inflammation also need to work on a cellular level.) These are very exciting substances that work:

- As functional foods.
- As nutritional supplements.
- As topical anti–aging therapies.

But these products are not the only tools at our disposal. Another indispensable method for fighting inflammation that delivers great results comes from the foods we eat. Sadly, many of our food choices are directly responsible for wrinkles, degenerative diseases, and accelerated aging. In this book, I introduce you to some important foods that may not be in your current diet, and reveal ten amazing and powerful superfoods, as well as herbs and spices, that you'll want to incorporate into your diet for their great anti-aging, health benefits. In addition to being rich in flavor, these foods are rich in nutrients and antioxidants. They will help you to not only live longer, but also look younger.

The neuropeptides, peptides, foods, and supplements introduced in these pages provide energy to the cells, helping them to function at optimum levels to keep you healthy and active well into middle age and beyond.

The Perricone Promise is my promise to you that these tools will deliver a rejuvenated face and body in just twenty-eight days. How can I make this claim? It's easy. Because all these foods, supplements, peptides, and neuropeptides, including the topical formulations, are *physiologic*—that is, they enable the body to utilize all their benefits. How? Because they work *with* the body and not against it, to accomplish their goals.

When we introduce a foreign substance (such as a pharmacologic agent) to the body, its benefit ends when we stop using the product or substance. In addition, there may be a host of negative side effects. However, when we deliver substances that are natural to the body, their therapeutic benefits increase each time, resulting in the ultimate strengthening and rejuvenating of all organ systems.

The Perricone Promise recommendations work synergistically, both internally and externally, to restore that youthful glow to your skin and vigor and vitality to your body. The side effects? The benefits keep increasing over time. Again, because the method of action is physiologic, our bodies do not develop resistance or immunity to the effects of these superfoods, neuropeptide technology, powerful anti-inflammatory supplements—and, best of all, topical treatments. You will start to see immediate benefits in as little as three days, with significant changes to face and body highly visible after the 28-Day Program. The longer you follow the program, the greater the physical and mental benefits.

Wishing you an exciting journey to greater health, beauty, and happiness.

NICHOLAS PERRICONE, M.D.
Madison, Connecticut
June 2004

PART I

EXPLAINING THE PROMISE

W hat are you doing for the next twenty-eight days? You could be taking ten years off the way you look and adding ten years on to your life by following the program laid out for you in the rest of this book.

In the first part of this book, you'll discover the breakthroughs on which this book is based. It's a breakthrough for me because it's the culmination of research I've been doing for years, research that provides irrefutable proof of the connections among inflammation, aging, and disease—and tells us what we can do about it.

You'll learn about one of the biggest breakthroughs in anti-aging medicine in years—protein-like substances in our bodies called peptides and neuropeptides. You'll also discover how they work both for us and against us, and how we can harness the positive power they offer to reduce harmful inflammation—and therefore begin to actually reverse the aging process.

It's not hard to do. Follow the three easy steps in part 2 (the foods, the supplements, the topicals) and put together for you in part 3 (the Perricone Program), and I promise that within twenty-eight days (or less), you'll look younger and feel healthier than you have in years.

The Perricone Promise

The world is so fast that there are days when the person who says it can't be done is interrupted by the person who is doing it.
—ANONYMOUS

The universe is full of magical things, patiently waiting for our wits to grow sharper.
—EDEN PHILLPOTTS

WHAT IF I WERE TO TELL YOU that we are on the threshold of a revolution that can reverse the signs of aging? And that with this book in hand, by following just *three simple steps,* you can start reaping these benefits today?

When I wrote *The Wrinkle Cure* and *The Perricone Prescription,* I introduced the Inflammation–Aging Connection—the concept that inflammation at the cellular level is the single most powerful cause of the signs of aging. That's not to mention the correlation between inflammation and such chronic diseases as arthritis, diabetes, Alzheimer's, cancer, and strokes.

The extensive research and the resulting solutions I introduced still hold true today, and thousands of people have reported how much better they look and feel after following my program.

I could have discontinued my research there. But I knew there was more to learn. I knew that if inflammation was at the root of aging, something deeper must be able to mediate that inflammation. That "something deeper" turns out to be the biggest breakthrough in anti-aging medicine in years: protein-like substances in our bodies called peptides and neuropeptides.

Peptides are compounds consisting of two or more amino acids (the building blocks of proteins), chained together by what is called a peptide bond.

Neuropeptides are peptides released by neurons (brain cells) as intercellular messengers. Some neuropeptides function as neurotransmitters, and others function as hormones.

Peptides and neuropeptides, like many substances in our bodies (think *cholesterol*) can work both for and against us. The good news is that by following the program in *The Perricone Promise,* you can dramatically increase the positive effects of anti-inflammatory peptides and neuropeptides and greatly decrease their negative influences.

As a result, you will experience dramatic changes not only in the way you look, but also in the way you feel. In just twenty-eight days, you can erase what seems like ten years from your face and body. With *The Perricone Promise,* you'll learn to help reverse the aging process and add many more youthful years to your life.

Look Better, Feel Better in Three Easy Steps

As a dermatologist, my primary interest and concern is how my patients look. Is your skin clear and healthy? Is your skin radiant and glowing, or is it dull and sallow? Is your skin heavily lined and wrinkled, or is it toned and supple? This concern does not stem from an obsession with youth or with looking like a model or film star. The answers to these questions are prime indicators of overall health. Your face and body are constant, visible monitors of how well or how poorly you are aging. Looking good and having a positive body image is not vanity; it is your road to a long, healthy, and happy life. This is one of the key reasons that I chose dermatology as a medical specialty—to be able to find new ways to achieve these highly visible goals regardless of chronological age.

My promise to you is that you can achieve these goals—looking younger and living longer—by following the three easy steps included in this book:

Step 1. DIET. A revolutionary nutritional program that includes the Ten Superfoods to help reduce inflammation and rejuvenate the skin and body.

Step 2. SUPPLEMENTS. In addition to eating well, these multi-purpose and highly effective nutritional supplements will increase production of the anti-inflammatory peptides and neuropeptides, your body's natural anti-aging weapons.

Step 3. TOPICALS. Working from the outside in, these newly for-mulated neuropeptide-based creams will have you looking younger almost instantly.

Throughout the rest of this book, you'll find ways of unleashing the power of neuropeptides to:

- Increase production of collagen and elastin.
- Repair scars and wrinkles.
- Increase circulation, resulting in breathtaking radiance and glow.
- Experience rapid wound repair.
- Develop a dewy, supple appearance to skin that you haven't seen since your teens.

But this book is not just about the way you look. By following this simple three-step program, you can rejuvenate not only your skin, but also your brain, your emotional state, and your overall health. Increasing the power of positive peptides can result in such diverse effects as:

- Decreased inflammation in every organ system.
- Increased efficiency of metabolism, resulting in cellular repair.
- Elevated mood.

- A strong and healthy heart that is resistant to disease.
- Denser bones as you age.
- Decreased risk of certain forms of cancer.
- Repair of the skin.
- Normalized metabolism for losing weight while retaining youth.
- A rejuvenated immune system.

The Brain–Beauty Connection

Each step I have taken in my career has led me to uncover secrets that go deep beneath the surface of the skin. When I began my research into peptides and neuropeptides, my goal was to help solve my patients' skin problems. I wanted to find ways to help them look healthier and younger.

How exciting, then, to discover that my research had much greater benefit than I ever imagined. It turns out that boosting the positive powers of peptides and neuropeptides will not only help you *look* healthier and younger, but actually help you maintain the health of every system and organ in your body—and even give you an edge on reversing the aging process. And it's all due to the Brain–Beauty Connection.

Prior to the discovery of neuropeptides, control of the brain and nervous system was thought to be accomplished through a complicated network of neurotransmitters (such as serotonin and dopamine), hormones (like adrenaline and cortisol), and enzymes.

Today, we know that matters are infinitely more complex. As brain researcher Dr. Steve Henricksen once put it, "We used to think the brain was like a computer. Now we think each cell is like a computer, a separate computer. And one single cell is like the whole brain."

If the brain is at all like a collection of integrated, high-speed computers, neuropeptides seem to form the electrochemical communications web that keeps them balanced and working in unison.

There are cells in the brain that produce various neuropeptides, and these neuropeptides do just about everything. They can be either pro-inflammatory or anti-inflammatory. They are responsible for many functions: They control our mood, energy levels, pain and pleasure reception, body weight, and ability to solve problems; they also form memories and regulate our immune system. These active little messengers in the brain actually turn on cellular function in the skin. (It's interesting to note that the immune system is an extension of the brain, and that the skin is an immune organ.)

Beauty Is Much More Than Skin Deep

When I was a medical student, we studied embryology. There I learned that three layers of tissue develop into every organ system in our bodies. One fact that particularly intrigued me was that the same layer of tissue that was responsible for the production of the brain also produced skin. That is why, when we eat a food or take a nutritional supplement that is therapeutic for the brain, the skin improves. This simple fact shaped much of my research into the role of peptides and neuropeptides in the Brain–Beauty Connection.

While manipulating the neuropeptides, neurotransmitters, and hormones that are in the brain to help create younger, more beautiful skin, increase longevity, and slow the aging process might seem more at home in a Michael Crichton or Robin Cook novel, believe me when I tell you that it is not only possible, but in fact the new reality.

Scientists now know that these neuropeptides, neurotransmitters, and hormones have a vast cellular communications system. Neuropeptides are nature's "cell" phones. There is a trio controlling every aspect of our bodies, using neuropeptides as their messengers. That is, the brain signals the thymus, which is the master gland of immunity (more about this in chapter 2); the thymus signals the skin; and the skin talks back to the brain. Every messenger has a *recipient* for its message. These recipients are known as *receptor sites*. Think of it as "cellular communication": The cells communicate in the same way as making a phone call from your phone (the messenger) to another phone, which is there to receive the call (the receptor site). There is no voice mail here—it is a world in which (for good or ill) every call is answered, instantly.

The message delivered at the receptor site depends upon the particular neuropeptide, neurotransmitter, or hormone making the call. If high levels of the potentially harmful neuropeptide Substance P (which you will also learn more about in chapter 2) are being released in the brain, for example, we will experience "psychic pain"—we will feel depressed and anxious. Substance P has receptor sites throughout the body, including in the skin, so the message or call sent to the receptors in the skin might be: "We're depressed. Let's turn on inflammation in our skin cells today."

The result? Accelerated aging of the skin through abnormal cell turnover, loss of radiance and tone.

So the brain sends messages to the skin. But remember, this "phone system" circuitry goes both ways. We now know that just by touching the skin, we can actually *change* the circuitry in our brain! This is an amazing concept if we take a minute to think about it. Usually we think it takes a powerful drug or surgical or therapeutic procedure of some sort to make any kind of significant change in the body or mind. However, studies have shown that just fifteen minutes of daily massage help premature infants gain weight faster, enabling them to leave the hospital sooner than their counterparts. The massaged babies are more relaxed, active, and alert. Six months later, they continue to be more advanced.

Studies in orphanages and hospitals repeatedly tell us that infants deprived of skin contact lose weight, become ill, and even die. Infants who are held cry less than those who are not, their immune systems are enhanced, and they handle stress more efficiently.

The need for touch continues throughout our lives. When diabetic children were massaged for a month, blood glucose levels decreased and they were able to reduce their medication levels. Asthmatic children had fewer attacks. Massage helped children with autism, severe burns, cancer, and arthritis. These are perfect illustrations of how neuropeptides can be activated in the brain from touch receptors in the skin. And the neuropeptides released, such as endorphins, send a healing, positive message to the brain.

NEUROPEPTIDES COME INTO THEIR OWN

I recently spoke with Jim Parker of the Do It Now Foundation, who shared with me some fascinating information on the world of neuropeptides back when they were first known as endorphins.

They were going to be the "magic bullets" of psychopharmacology, miraculous chemical keys to unlock the secrets of pleasure and pain, joy and sorrow, memory, intelligence, and behavior.

They were supposed to explain everything from falling in love to falling asleep, and a full understanding of their actions and effects was going to cure drug addiction and mental illness, regulate mood and appetite, and even heighten creativity and sexual response.

They were the endorphins, the internally produced morphine-like substances responsible for an array of drug-like effects in the body, and for a while after their 1975 discovery, everyone wanted to speculate about them.

But the euphoria didn't last. Life got complicated as research findings grew confusing, then contradictory. As the number of identified endorphins grew from month to month, and scientists' understanding of their many effects broadened, they became known as endogenous opioids, and finally neuropeptides, of which endorphins form a small subcategory.

Investigators continued to look hard and long at the powerful new body of chemicals and quietly went about the difficult work of figuring them out—or at least figuring out a way to figure them out.

In the process, they linked them with a vast array of physical and emotional problems—as both possible causes and potential cures—and the prognosis is now good for at least some of the promised early magic bullets to hit their mark. In human terms, for the millions of people afflicted with a wide range of problems from alcoholism and obesity to chronic pain and schizophrenia, the study of neuropeptides holds great promise.

Botox? Notox!

One of the great joys of practicing dermatology is seeing immediate, visible effects when the right treatment is applied to a particular condition. This has been a great motivator for me throughout my career, and it continues to provide the inspiration for spending many hours in the laboratory looking for that next miracle ingredient that can truly deliver results to the skin.

For far too long, the beauty and skin care industry has focused on the look and feel of a product—its packaging and its perfume, as opposed to genuine efficacy. Since I first introduced topical formulations containing highly active ingredients such as alpha lipoic acid (ALA) and dimethylaminoethanol (DMAE), retailers have had a hard time keeping their shelves stocked with these products. A new generation of women and men is controlling the marketplace—a generation that not only wants but actually *demands* products that work overtime to keep them as young looking and as vital as possible. I think this is an excellent development, because it has now involved many major corporations in serious research aimed toward resolving the problems of aging skin.

However, there is a somewhat alarming trend toward obtaining serious (and very costly) surgical procedures at a younger and younger age. Just turn on the TV and you will see some young woman, still in her teens, vying for radical surgery to turn herself into a clone of the current hot actress, model, or singer. America seems to be gripped by manic, radical makeover madness. According to a *New York Times* article, "A Lovelier You, With Off-the-Shelf Parts" by Alex Kuczynski (May 2, 2004), Americans underwent 8.3 million cosmetic surgery procedures in 2003, an increase of 12 percent over the previous year.

In addition to all the surgery, new fillers designed to plump up facial lines are being rushed to market. Use of Botox, a neurotoxin (*neuro* means "nerve"; *toxin* means "poison") that paralyzes muscles to smooth out wrinkles and expression lines, is rampant. The Kuczynski article reports that the number of nonsurgical procedures, such as Botox, rose 22 percent over the previous year to 6.4 million. These products offer a quick fix, but there are questions about their long-term safety, questions that won't be answered for years to come.

My ongoing goal is to find the Notox solution to signs and symptoms of aging on the face and in the body. This has led me to develop what might be termed the next generation of skin and body care—the peptides and neuropeptides.

Reversing the Aging Process

In *The Wrinkle Cure* and *The Perricone Prescription,* I introduced a major theme of my research: the Inflammation–Disease–Aging Connection. Because inflammation is a great contributor to accelerated aging, it has been an important focus of my ongoing scientific research. And we now know that neuropeptides and peptides play an important role in mediating inflammation.

For those of you who may not be familiar with the Inflammation–Aging Connection, here is a quick review.

Inflammation exists as a spectrum ranging from the highly visible, such as bright red sunburn, to the invisible. It is this invisible inflammation that I am referring to when I use the term *inflammation.* You can't see it and you can't feel it. This invisible inflammation (also called micro-inflammation) exists in all of our cells and is responsible for their eventual breakdown. It is responsible for the aging process that gives us wrinkled, sagging skin as well as age-related diseases as diverse as Alzheimer's, diabetes, cancer, cardiovascular disease, arthritis, and the autoimmune diseases.

Simply put, if we want to decrease our risk for age-related diseases and decelerate the aging process, then we need to control inflammation. And we can do that best by controlling two essential lifestyle elements: *diet* and *stress.*

DIET AND AGING: THE SUGAR CONNECTION

There are many causes of the inflammation–aging process, but I believe the primary cause is diet. Foods that we eat can either be pro-inflammatory (they provoke an inflammatory response) or anti-inflammatory (they suppress the inflammatory response). Pro-inflammatory foods are those that cause a rapid rise in blood sugar, resulting in the release of insulin into the bloodstream. The chief culprits in the pro-inflammatory arena are sugar and foods that quickly convert to sugar in the bloodstream, such as potatoes, breads, pastries, juice, chips, and rice cakes.

We have to understand and accept this simple but painful fact of life: Sugar can be toxic. Ingesting sugar causes a rise in blood sugar, resulting in a burst of inflammatory chemicals that spread throughout our bodies. Even worse, from a dermatological point of view, is that sugar can permanently attach to the collagen present in our skin and other parts of our body through a process known as *glycation*. Where the sugar attaches, there is a little mechanism creating inflammation, and that attachment becomes a source of inflammation in its own right. This inflammation produces enzymes that break down collagen, resulting in wrinkles. In addition to creating inflammation, glycation results in the cross-linking of our collagen, making it stiff and inflexible—somewhat like a soft, supple leather boot that has been left out in the rain and is now hard and stiff and brittle.

But it's not only glycation of the skin we have to worry about. The overconsumption of sugar produces stiff sugar–protein bonds, which accumulate throughout our bodies as we get older. The sugar or glucose molecule "glues" itself to our collagen, as well as to our veins, arteries, ligaments, bones—even our brains! We then suffer from stiff joints, hardened arteries, failing organs—basically, sugar contributes to the deterioration of every bodily function.

It's easy to see why we must avoid foods that cause elevated levels of sugar. *The Perricone Promise* provides many excellent food choices, recipes, and meal plans that will prevent this age-accelerating, dietary inflammation.

STRESS AND AGING: THE ANXIETY CONNECTION

A second very important mediator of inflammation is stress. There are two kinds of stress—*physical* and *psychic*—and both cause inflammation. Physical stress can be caused by trauma, wounds, even the stretching of the skin from normal gravity. There is pretty good evidence that the gravity pulling on your skin when you simply get out of bed in the morning can result in an inflammatory response in your skin (my son often used this line to avoid school).

Mental or psychic stress can be just as detrimental as physical stress. When you are stressed (regardless of the cause), you produce neuropeptides that exert a negative effect on your brain by triggering the production of cortisol, a hormone that can have dire consequences for your health when produced in large amounts.

Cortisol is made by the adrenal glands, which sit above the kidneys. Cortisol is needed to activate the body when it is under stress, enabling us to survive physically dangerous situations through what is known as the fight-or-flight syndrome. The release of cortisol allows our muscles to be fueled for action. Cortisol is an emergency hormone called into play in desperate situations.

However, when a high level of cortisol circulates in the body for long periods of time, it is toxic to our organ systems. It will actually destroy brain cells, elevate our blood sugar (resulting in diabetes), cause damage to the immune system (making us more susceptible to infection and cancer), elevate our blood pressure, decalcify our bones, and thin our skin.

The more stress you're under, the greater the amount of cortisol produced. These stress-related neuropeptides and hormones also send messages to the immune system, effectively shutting it down. And that is not all. The same neuropeptides send signals directly to the skin and produce an inflammatory response. The more stress you have in your life, the greater the chance that inflammation will occur somewhere in or on your body.

Luckily, the two major causes of inflammation—diet and stress—are also the most controllable. In *The Perricone Promise,* you will discover a variety of strategies to suppress the release of pro-inflammatory neuropeptides (the "bad" guys), while encouraging the production of anti-inflammatory neuropeptides (the "good" guys).

- In Step 1, I will talk about diet and much of the very latest research on foods that have great anti-inflammatory powers. You will learn, for instance, a color-coordinated system for choosing foods that have the highest amounts of natural peptide boosters and anti-inflammatories.
- In Step 2, you will learn which nutritional supplements have significant anti-inflammatory activity and be introduced to special polysaccharide peptide "foods" that have great therapeutic potential for the skin, body, and brain.
- In Step 3, I will add the topical products that include the latest scientific breakthrough on the anti-aging/anti-inflammation front. Research over the past twenty years has uncovered the critical role of small, hormone-like protein fragments called *thymic peptides,* which exert beneficial anti-aging, anti-inflammatory, healing, and anti-cancer effects in the body. You'll learn which topical products contain these healing substances and how to apply them effectively.

To find out more about why peptides and neuropeptides are critical to the anti-aging/anti-inflammation process, read the next chapter. It will help you understand how and why the foods, supplements, and topicals I'm recommending will restore your looks and health. In the meantime, I urge you to start Step 1 of the program so you don't spend one more unnecessary day prematurely aging your body and mind.

2 The Science Behind the Promise

There is a single light of science, and to brighten it anywhere is to brighten it everywhere.

— ISAAC ASIMOV

WHERE DO PEPTIDES AND NEUROPEPTIDES ORIGINATE? This chapter will give you some background on the organs and systems that produce peptides and neuropeptides, introduce you to a peptide (or two) that has great therapeutic promise, and warn you about another peptide that is the source of many of the mind and body's aches, pains, and degenerative diseases.

As mentioned in chapter 1, there is a vast, intricate, and highly efficient communications network of peptide and neuropeptide messengers circulating throughout our bodies whose complexity far exceeds our most sophisticated technology. These messengers are extremely important. They have taught us that it is not just the major neurotransmitters such as serotonin, dopamine, and norepinephrine that control our moods and our brain. We now know that there is a fine tuning performed by neurotransmitters and an even *finer tuning* performed by neuropeptides. We also know that this vast intracellular network, made up of the endocrine and nervous systems, controls the rate at which our brain, skin, and organ systems age.

That's what makes the Perricone Promise so exciting. Once we know the cause of something, we can design a therapeutic intervention. Of course, we can't *cure* aging. As with most other degenerative diseases, however, we can do everything in our power to slow down its destructive effects. That's what you're doing by following the three-step program in this book—you're utilizing every tool available (some as ancient as food and some as new as thymic extracts) to combat your body's enemies.

Setting Your Body in Motion

As I said earlier, some messengers function as neurotransmitters, and others function as hormones. Organs that produce hormones are called endocrine (*en*-doh-kryn) glands. (While the brain and kidneys also produce hormones, they are not considered endocrine organs, since this is a minor part of their function.) In Greek, *hormone* means "to set in motion"; hormones are made by endocrine glands to control or "set in motion" another part of the body.

The endocrine system works hand in hand with the nervous system. In fact, the endocrine and nervous systems are so closely linked that they are more accurately viewed as a single *neuroendocrine* system, which performs several critical tasks:

- Maintains the body's internal steady state or homeostasis (nutrition, metabolism, excretion, and water and salt balances).
- Reacts to stimuli from outside the body.
- Regulates growth, development, and reproduction.
- Produces, uses, and stores energy.

The neuroendocrine system is designed to ensure each individual's safety from external or internal threats, and the hormones most responsible for this task are called stress hormones.

LIVE TO FIGHT ANOTHER DAY...

The body produces two kinds of hormones: steroids and peptides.

Steroidal hormones such as testosterone, estrogen, and cortisol, are produced by the adrenal cortex, ovaries, and testes. These hormones affect reproduction, thereby helping ensure the survival of the species.

Peptide hormones are manufactured in nerve cell structures of the hypothalamus (the part of the brain most involved in the regulation of hormone secretion) and bathe the pituitary gland. The thymus also produces peptide-like hormones, which initiate a cascade of biochemical reactions that produce effects throughout the body. These hormones facilitate the functioning of all the organs.

Haunted by "Death" Hormones

The neuroendocrine system is under particular strain in today's world. Not only does it serve as the foundation of our emotional lives, but it must also deal with threats from our external environment. The neuroendocrine system affects us even before we are born: Maternal stress during pregnancy is thought to have an effect on the formation of the critical hypothalamic–pituitary axis. Childhood experiences can affect our behavior in later life, and the hormonal system bears the brunt of it. Children growing up in dysfunctional homes may become "adrenaline junkies," trying to re-create the patterns they became accustomed to in childhood as well as the highly charged emotions they experienced exacerbated by elevated blood levels of adrenaline and cortisol. Chronically elevated levels of those hormones can eventually produce autoimmune syndromes, memory loss, chronic fatigue syndrome, and cancer, as well as accelerating the aging process.

As we grow older, secretion of many hormones declines and their effectiveness (compared unit to unit) is reduced because the cellular receptors that accept individual hormones become less responsive. Unfortunately, the ones that decline are the "youth hormones" (growth hormones, sex steroids), while the "death hormones" (cortisol and insulin) continue to rise. In addition, ubiquitous "endocrine disrupters"—environmental chemicals such as pesticides and plastics—can bind to target cells' receptors and block hormones from gaining entry.

As stress levels increase, levels of the death hormones also increase, causing systemwide damage with results like emotional chaos, memory loss, weight gain—and, of course, inflammation throughout the body. Even drinking coffee can raise cortisol levels and keep them elevated throughout the day. Too much cortisol can produce extensive biological damage and is a leading cause of premature aging. So a squabble with your spouse over a cup of coffee at breakfast combined with a spurt of road rage on the way to work will conspire to ensure that you are anxious, forgetful, depressed, and packing on the pounds for the next twenty-four-hour period!

Here It Comes to Save the Day!

One of the ways the body counteracts the damage done by stress hormones and human behavioral factors (poor diet, too much caffeine, not enough sleep or exercise) is by repairing the immune system.

Tucked behind the sternum between the lungs is the *thymus,* the master gland and Mighty Mouse of the immune system. Small though it is, we cannot talk about the overall health of the body, under stressful conditions or otherwise, without discussing the thymus. This long-overlooked gland only began to garner serious scientific attention in the 1980s, when researchers realized that it is the key to a healthy immune system.

The thymus gland produces thymic peptides and thymic hormones. Thymic peptides:

- Are directly responsible for the maturation of *T cells*—white blood cells activated by the thymus that play a major role in the body's immune response.
- Directly influence other immune functions such as antibody production.
- Are fundamental to the integration and proper interaction among the immune, endocrine, and central nervous systems.

THYMIC MENOPAUSE

The thymus continues to develop after birth and reaches maximum size during puberty. After puberty, gradual shrinking of the thymus, called *involution*, occurs steadily. By age thirty, the thymus gland has typically decreased its mass by two-thirds and its T cell content by 90 percent. By age sixty, functional thymic tissue has almost completely disappeared, potentially compromising the integrity of the aging immune system.

This inevitable weakening of the immune system is a natural decline known as *immunosenescence*. It is this "thymic menopause" that affects both sexes and causes an increased susceptibility to infections, autoimmune diseases, and cancer as we age.

The Anti-Aging Promise of Thymic Peptides

It is the thymus gland that, like a thermostat, controls the immune system. When foreign invaders arrive, such as infections or tumors, bacteria or viruses, thymic production goes up. It goes down in order to prevent autoimmune diseases (when the body's defenses against infection are turned against the body itself).

Because aging is a progressive, degenerative disease, I can tell you that I've made an extensive study of the thymus and how it might reverse many of the signs of aging:

- Studies have shown the beneficial effects of liquid thymus extracts on the structure and function of livers in aging animals. In addition, the liver and spleen function of the treated animals did not deteriorate with age.

- Similar studies have shown that thymic peptides decrease the levels of oxidized fatty acids in the brain and spleen tissue of adult animals, and significantly increase their longevity.

- In addition, we know that thymus gland hormones increase the quantity and quality of the body's T cells, and T cells secrete human growth hormone (HGH). Thymic peptides also stimulate the pituitary gland to release HGH. Human growth hormone is the true "youth" hormone. It builds muscle, increases the vitality of the body's organ systems, and decreases the levels of the stress hormone cortisol. It would be helpful to increase the amount of HGH the body produces; however, there are many questions and concerns about the safety profile and side effects of administering HGH directly into the system. Studies have shown that a much safer route is to use thymic peptides to trigger the body's own release of HGH from the pituitary gland.

The conclusion is obvious: *Not only do thymic peptides enhance immunity, but they also slow and even reverse the process of organ aging.*

The Therapeutic Promise of Thymic Extracts

The knowledge that thymic peptides directly influence immune function led scientists to ask how they could be extracted and used to treat immune system problems. Numerous animal tests and a limited number of clinical trials have produced highly positive results and persuaded most medical researchers that thymus extracts possess real potential for treating a wide range of conditions:

- Autoimmune conditions (such as lupus and rheumatoid arthritis).
- Cancers (breast, lung, larynx, head/neck, leukemia, Hodgkin's disease, and non-Hodgkin's lymphoma).

- Chronic infections (viral, fungal, parasitical).
- Cornea damage.
- Hepatitis B and other liver conditions.
- Herpes simplex and zoster.
- Immunodeficiency conditions (such as AIDS).
- Inflammatory skin diseases (like psoriasis and atopic eczema).
- Postsurgical infections.
- Respiratory infections.
- Severe and chronic respiratory allergies.

They can also accelerate wound healing, and have shown promise as agents to enhance the effectiveness of anti-cancer radiation and chemotherapy, and decrease their adverse side effects.

Because, in essence, a wrinkle can be considered a wound, the amazing wound-healing properties of the thymic peptides inspired me to explore their use in reversing many of the signs of aging. As always, I approached the problem from a holistic view, first to see what effect they might have systemically if taken internally, and also to examine the effects topical preparations might have.

The results have generally been very encouraging, regardless of whether the thymus extracts were administered orally or by injection, which is why I have developed my healthy peptide nutritional program as well as a line of thymic peptide supplements (both of which are described in detail later in the book). Catherine's story shows the power of the thymic peptides in action.

Catherine's Story

If you want to know how increasing healthy thymic peptide function can improve how you look and feel, consider Catherine's story.

I first met Catherine during Fashion Week in New York City. Even though it was early fall, the temperatures were hovering in the low nineties. All of Bryant Park was covered in tents, reminiscent of a Renaissance fair.

I had created special Fashion Week Survival Kits consisting of little cans of salmon, nuts, blueberries, and bottled springwater for the models and designers, and many of them approached me throughout the day to say thanks. Such was the case with Catherine, a model who, though extremely beautiful, looked exhausted. I suggested to Catherine that she take a short rest and handed her a bottle of water.

"Thanks, Dr. Perricone," Catherine said, graciously accepting a seat out of the hot sun. "I don't know how I am going to get through the rest of the day! I feel like I could sleep for a week," she added, nervously searching for a cigarette.

Like many models, Catherine chain-smoked and drank copious amounts of coffee. And she was burning the proverbial candle at both ends, enjoying the rounds of parties and club-hopping that go with the modeling territory. "Usually I have energy to spare," she confided. "But I don't know how I am going to get through the rest of this week. To make matters worse, it seems that every time I turn around I'm coming down with a cold, or the flu, or an allergy attack."

Catherine's smoking, high stress levels, excessive coffee drinking, and lack of sleep were keeping high levels of cortisol circulating in her blood. She was doing a great job of upsetting the delicate balance of her endocrine and nervous systems. She appeared to be functioning on pure adrenaline.

I told Catherine I didn't need to explain the long-term dangers of her lifestyle, and continued that she could start to counteract these negative effects immediately. While I couldn't get her to stop smoking then and there, she was willing to think about cutting back on both cigarettes and coffee.

For now I suggested she try to get more sleep. "That alone will help you get through the week with energy to spare," I said.

Since sleep is so important to rejuvenation, it is essential that you do whatever you can to enhance the sleep experience. A few alcoholic beverages in the evening may initially make you drowsy, but very soon the alcohol precipitates a systemic burst of norepinephrine—a hormone that increases as a result of excitement or stress. Hours after taking a drink, a burst of norepinephrine occurs and causes you to come back to consciousness. This was happening with Catherine, who would enjoy two or three cosmopolitans on her nights out, fall asleep, and then wake several hours later, resulting in a very poor night's sleep.

"Caffeine in the late afternoon and evening can also interfere with your sleep patterns," I told her. "In addition, before going to bed, you should avoid any food that will cause a rapid rise in your blood sugar; it will interfere with growth hormone production, robbing you of this essential anti-aging hormone. And if you exercise at night, do it at least four hours before bedtime." Catherine admitted that dancing was a big part of her nightly partying. It was no wonder she looked so tired!

I was not suggesting that Catherine never drink, never party, or never dance again—just that she shouldn't do it every night.

In order to counteract all these negative things, I asked Catherine to just promise to eat one serving of salmon and fresh salad a day and try to follow the Perricone Promise 28-Day Program— although I knew this wasn't realistic. I also gave her a box of my Total Skin and Body supplements, because I knew that she would not forget to take them. She was actually excited about trying the special thymic peptide supplements, which would help balance and regulate the various systems in her body that she was busily driving into a state of dysfunction. I have specially formulated these supplements to also help support immune function and felt this would help Catherine be less susceptible to colds, flu, and allergies.

About a month later, I ran into Catherine at a fund-raiser. I was immediately impressed with how healthy she looked. "Dr. Perricone," she enthused, "I want to thank you. I feel really really wonderful. I haven't been getting sick, my energy levels are great, and best of all, that stressed-out, anxious feeling is gone." Catherine was taking the vitamins and thymic peptide supplements faithfully and felt that they had really made a significant difference. She hadn't stopped the use of coffee and cigarettes but had cut back considerably, and was much more conscious of her nutritional intake. "I still enjoy the occasional cosmopolitan," she laughed, "but I am sleeping much better."

Our bodies are finely tuned to a delicate balance, and I believe that in addition to following the anti-inflammatory diet and lifestyle, peptides and neuropeptides in the correct formulations can help us maintain this critical balance. Thymic peptides in particular show great promise in stimulating the immune system, in wound healing, and in providing multiple disease-preventing and anti-aging benefits.

The Bad News Is . . .

Chemicals in the body, whether they are neuropeptides, peptides, neurotransmitters, or hormones, can produce dual effects—some positive and some negative. Consider, for example, the hormone estrogen. Estrogen helps keep our skin healthy and supple and our bones strong. However, an excess of estrogen may be a contributing factor in PMS, whose symptoms can range from body aches and fluid retention to migraine headaches and fatigue, from irritability and mood swings to suicidal and homicidal thoughts and actions.

This is also true of neuropeptides and peptides, which can exert either an anti-inflammatory or a pro-inflammatory effect on the body. One such neuropeptide in particular, known as *Substance P,* exists in various organs in our body and plays a significant role in many mental and physical functions. On the positive side, Substance P helps widen blood vessels and tighten the intestines and other smooth muscles. It also plays a part in the release of saliva and urine. On the negative side, Substance-P-triggered inflammation in the skin makes us wrinkled and gives us acne. Even worse, Substance P has a direct link to such seemingly unrelated chronic, progressive concerns as aging, depression, obesity, alcoholism, and pain.

Substance P was discovered around 1930. At the time, scientists had no idea what it did. Eventually, they learned that Substance P is involved in the transmission of pain impulses. In fact, it was discovered that Substance P creates sort of a chronic pain-delivery system that travels from the spinal cord to the brain. Substance P is also released by certain nerve endings in the skin so that when the skin is traumatized, Substance P is released, and that's when you feel the pain.

When Substance P is released into your skin, it not only delivers pain signals but also creates an inflammatory cascade throughout the body. In chapter 7, you'll discover how Substance P's harmful effects become visible on the skin. Right now, let's look at how Substance P's brain–pain continuum causes vital brain cells to go haywire.

SUBSTANCE P AND THE BRAIN–BEAUTY CONNECTION

Substance P is synthesized and released in many organ systems, including the brain. The release of Substance P in the brain cannot cause physical pain. This is because the brain has *no* pain receptors in it at all. In fact, surgery can be performed on the brain without anesthesia. However, what it does cause is *psychic* pain. This psychic or mental pain is manifested as anxiety and depression. Scientists have administered Substance P to volunteers so that brain levels of this neuropeptide increased above normal. These volunteers reported feelings of anxiety and depression very soon after the neuropeptide was administered.

Substance P is involved with the perceptions of both pleasure and pain. Studies have shown that if you reduce Substance P, you reduce the stress that's linked to pain. If you reduce the stress, you reduce the inflammation. If you reduce the inflammation, you decelerate the aging process. But there's more.

Studies conducted by Stephen P. Hunt of University College, London, showed that Substance P is found in parts of the brain associated with the motivational properties of comforting "rewards" such as food and recreational drugs. Reduce the Substance P, and you reduce the cravings for the kinds of rewards that destroy our health, create emotional chaos, and make us look and feel years older than we should.

THE INCREDIBLE SHRINKING BRAIN

When Substance P is released, it is accompanied by additional amino acids such as glutamate and aspartate, which result in a state known as *excitotoxicity*. Glutamate, a neurotransmitter, is essential for learning and both short-term and long-term memory. Glutamate normally exists in extracellular fluid in very, very small concentrations. When these concentrations begin to rise, neurons (our brain cells) begin to fire abnormally. At higher concentrations, the cells undergo the specialized process of cell death known as excitotoxicity; that is, they are excited to death. The deaths of these cells can cause a variety of neurodegenerative disorders, including ALS (commonly known as Lou Gehrig's disease) and Alzheimer's disease.

FOOD ADDITIVES, ARTIFICIAL SWEETENERS, AND EXCITOTOXICITY

A group of compounds called excitotoxins plays a critical role in the development of many neurological disorders, including migraines, seizures, infections, abnormal neural development, certain endocrine disorders, neuropsychiatric disorders, learning disorders in children, AIDS dementia, episodic violence, Lyme borreliosis, hepatic encephalopathy, specific types of obesity, and especially the neurodegenerative diseases such as amyotrophic lateral sclerosis (ALS), Parkinson's disease, Alzheimer's disease, Huntington's disease, and olivopontocerebellar degeneration. An enormous amount of both clinical and experimental evidence has accumulated over the past decade supporting these findings. Yet the immediate and long-term danger to the public caused by the practice of allowing various excitotoxins to be added to the food supply—including monosodium glutamate (MSG), hydrolyzed vegetable protein, and aspartame—goes unheeded.

> **The amount of these neurotoxins added to our food has increased enormously since their introduction. These are substances, usually acidic amino acids, that react with specialized receptors in the brain in such a way as to lead to destruction of certain types of neurons. Glutamate, the neurotransmitter most commonly used by the brain, is one of the most commonly known excitotoxins. MSG is the sodium salt of glutamate. You should therefore avoid MSG, as well as aspartame and food additives such as yeast extract, textured protein, soy protein extract, and the like, all of which are excitotoxins. What's the best way to do this? Buy your foods in their most natural, unprocessed state and add your own fresh or dried herbs and spices.**

It is now known that when Substance P, which can cause depression, is released along with glutamate, the resulting excitotoxicity has additional negative effects on our brain cells. The overexcitement of the neurons combined with the depression ultimately results not only in the death of the brain cells but also in the actual *shrinking* of our brain. When we are mentally stressed, whether it is from an argument with our spouse or worry about our financial situation, Substance P is released in the brain, with potentially disastrous effects.

And Now for the Good News

With all this talk about the harmful effects of that insidious villain Substance P, by now you must be thinking, *What's a body to do?* That's what the rest of this chapter—and the rest of this book—is all about. There is research currently going on and some specific steps you can take to reduce the negative effects of Substance P.

Excitotoxicity reducers. We now know that traditional anti-depressants can decrease excitotoxicity caused by Substance P. Recently, several nutrients have been found that significantly reduce excitotoxicity, including pycnogenol, acetyl-L-carnitine, and combinations of coenzyme Q10 and niacinamide. Preliminary experiments using natural Substance P blockers in the brain resulted in a marked calming of anxiety without having to resort to the current crop of tranquilizers and their resultant side effects. Other clinical trials using Substance P blockers are also promising in terms of alleviating depression; Substance P blockers appear to be more effective in some cases of depression than traditional anti-depressants such as Prozac and Paxil.

Substance P blockers. Scientists are now conducting several studies using chemicals that have been found to block or suppress high levels of Substance P. One of these blockers is currently in use: capsaicin, the ingredient in hot peppers that makes them "hot." It is a natural Substance P blocker and can be taken as a supplement, eaten as a food in the form of hot peppers, salsa, and other similar foods, or applied topically. Capsaicin cream can be used for the chronic pain of shingles, and for the inflammation seen in acne and eczema. It's not a magic bullet, but many patients have found it very helpful. More information about capsaicin can be found in chapter 4.

Stress relievers. As you have seen throughout these first two chapters, high levels of stress increase production of harmful hormones and neuropeptides, including Substance P. To counteract these high levels, you need to find ways of counteracting the stress—which is, after all, impossible to avoid completely. Try instituting a program of moderate exercise. Exercise of almost any kind has a powerful, positive, anti-inflammatory effect on all your cells. And exercise is a wonderful tension reliever. Just remember, moderation is the key. Exercise that is too strenuous will have a pro-inflammatory effect on the body. You should also reserve time during the day (a good time is right before going to bed) for quiet and meditation. Take this opportunity to empty your mind of all the details of your day—good and bad— or to pray, if that is your belief. A companion animal can also be a wonderful loving, nonjudgmental stress reliever. These simple acts can have lifelong benefits.

Neuropeptide Y. Scientists are looking into ways to boost the production of Neuropeptide Y, sometimes called the "calm and courageous" peptide. When Neuropeptide Y is released in the brain, it inhibits anxiety and depression, and can also increase appetite and improve the memory. Neuropeptide Y's other effects on the body are the constriction of blood vessels, the regulation of body temperature and blood pressure, and control of the release of the sex hormones.

One discovery that has particularly intrigued physicians resulted from a study of post-traumatic stress disorder (PTSD). Researchers noted that PTSD is virtually never seen in Special Forces—SEALs or Rangers or any of the Special Ops soldiers—who are subjected to extreme mental, emotional, and physical stress conditions on an ongoing basis. Apparently, Special Forces soldiers have higher levels of Neuropeptide Y in their central nervous systems. And even though physical and psychological stress can reduce these levels significantly, Special Forces soldiers show a rapid return to normal levels of Neuropeptide Y after exposure to stress. Regular soldiers *do not*—hence their much greater susceptibility to PTSD. Scientists believe that it is the high levels of Neuropeptide Y that make the Special Forces soldiers resistant to PTSD and also account for their exceptional courage and calmness while in combat.

Obviously, Neuropeptide Y has the opposite effect of Substance P, whose elevated levels contribute to anxiety, depression, fear, and nervousness. The good news is that the same elements that suppress levels of Substance P also elevate levels of Neuropeptide Y. Because we all need to be "Super Soldiers" to cope with life in today's world, throughout these chapters the Perricone Promise will provide strategies to help us maintain elevated levels of Neuropeptide Y while suppressing excess levels of Substance P.

Neuropeptides: The DNA of Consciousness?

One reason I am so excited about the anti-aging prospects of neuropeptides is that there is so much still to be learned. It remains to be seen just how long it will take to fully uncover the as-yet-unsolved mysteries of the neuropeptides and, through them, learn the secrets of the brain, personality, and consciousness itself.

As work with neuropeptides has widened steadily over the years—

beyond analgesia and other drug states to memory, sensation, appetite, and emotion—researchers have come to grasp the immense significance of the task before them: deciphering the codes of consciousness. And as the neuropeptides have emerged as the neurobiological equivalent of DNA, researchers have glimpsed the incredible potential of the corkscrew chains and spirals of amino acids permeating the brain and central nervous system. These chemical clusters are not, scientists have come to recognize, merely an artifact of thought or sensation or emotion; rather, they *are* the thought or sensation or emotion—or all of it our brains ever know. It's the ultimate reduction or clarification of Descartes' famous argument: "My brain is full of neuropeptides; therefore I am."

Exciting research is ongoing, and I am optimistic that as we unlock the secrets of neuropeptides, we can look forward to enhanced memory, longer lives, and expanded emotional well-being.

Some secrets have already been unlocked and are the basis of the Perricone Promise 28-Day Program. In part 2 of this book, you'll learn exciting new discoveries about food, supplements, and topical creams that will help you look younger and live healthier for many years to come.

PART II

THE THREE STEPS

The basic concepts in this book—the Inflammation–Aging–Disease Connections—are the same concepts I've been talking about for years. What's different is that *The Perricone Promise* goes deeper than ever before into the very root of the inflammation process: the role the peptides and neuropeptides play. This book concentrates on whole-body anti-aging; it's not just about looking younger, but also about living longer.

The way to target these peptides and neuropeptides, reduce their negative effects, and boost their positive powers is to aim at them from every angle possible—from the outside in and from the inside out.

It starts, of course, with food. How you age depends on what you eat. The foods you consume can work to inhibit inflammation, or they can promote it. Chapters 3, 4, and 5 will help you decide which are the healthiest foods (including the Ten Superfoods!) to choose to reduce inflammation and rejuvenate the skin and body.

Chapter 6 will introduce you to supplements that are revolutionary weapons in the anti-aging armament: the polysaccharides—a new way to help increase the body's energy from as deep inside the body as you can get, the cells themselves. Chapter 7 continues the process by introducing you to a number of multipurpose and highly effective nutritional supplements that will increase production of the anti-inflammatory peptides and neuropeptides, your body's natural anti-aging weapons.

The last chapter in this section introduces you to the topicals. Working from the outside in, these newly formulated neuropeptide-based creams will have you looking younger almost instantly.

The purpose of these chapters is to give you the background you need to make the right decisions for a longer, healthier life. Knowledge is power, and the knowledge you'll gain throughout the rest of this book will keep you looking and feeling better throughout the rest of your life.

STEP ONE

THE FOODS

3 Rainbow Foods
Where the Pot of Gold Is the Rainbow

I cannot pretend to be impartial about the colors. I rejoice with the brilliant ones, and am genuinely sorry for the poor browns.
—SIR WINSTON CHURCHILL

JUST AS WINSTON CHURCHILL found his greatest pleasure painting with brilliant colors, you will enjoy great health and culinary benefits when you choose foods imbued with the myriad hues of the rainbow. However, Sir Winston need not feel sorry for the "poor browns." These brown pigments, for example, are what give nuts and a wide variety of beans and legumes their great phytonutrient activity. It's a very convenient coincidence that health-promoting capacity follows color—and it stems from a serendipitous circumstance. Plant pigments don't just add color to fruits, vegetables, and certain seafood: They also serve as the top dietary sources of disease-preventive phytonutrients and anti-aging, anti-inflammatory antioxidants. Mother Nature makes it easy to choose her most healthful fare: Simply favor the most vivid and deeply colored artist's palette of plant and sea foods!

Brett's Story

I recently had the honor of speaking at an international conference on the future of beauty and health. My topic was the intrinsic relationship of inner health to outer beauty. I discussed at length the role of diet, supplements, and topical therapies and how they all work synergistically to achieve this goal.

After the lecture, I was introduced to Brett, an attractive brunette who had just celebrated her fortieth birthday. Brett worked for an international cosmetics company, and after chatting a few minutes she said: "I really enjoyed your lecture, Dr. Perricone, and I'm fascinated to think that certain foods can really have an impact on beauty. Just about every woman I know, myself included, eats with weight in mind—not complexion." She continued, "But I can't help notice that my skin could use some major help. I think that I'm a prime candidate for your program!" Brett's skill and the liberal use of her firm's products enabled her to disguise it, but upon close inspection I could see that her skin had lost the fresh radiance of youth and appeared dull and dry. She had also developed fine lines and wrinkles around the eyes and mouth.

Brett was at a very vulnerable age—choices she made now would come to haunt her (or delight her) as she approached fifty. "The late thirties and early forties are important times in our lives," I explained. "Women especially have to deal with hormonal and other changes. Now is the time to really pay attention to what you eat because your diet and lifestyle can either slow down the aging process or speed it up. And the first place this is visible is the face."

I asked Brett to give me an example of what she ate. Much to my horror, Brett admitted that rice cakes—especially the white cheddar flavor—were pretty much her dietary staple. "I live alone and just can't get excited about whipping up a gourmet meal for one. However," she added, "if I thought I could eat 'real' food and not gain weight, believe me, Dr. Perricone, I would!"

I told Brett that she might want to rethink her eating philosophy, because this innocent-looking little snack food is quickly converted to sugar. Why? Rice and corn have a high glycemic index

(GI), making these foods pro-inflammatory. And when they are "puffed," their GI really skyrockets off the charts—in fact, their glycemic index is actually higher than that of table sugar! Eating a rice or corn cake generates the insulin response that causes us to store, rather than burn, fat. Brett admitted that even though she ate very few calories, she had a difficult time losing weight. "That's because the rice cakes cause an insulin release—which results in the storage of body fat," I explained.

Fat *and* Wrinkled?

If this was not enough of a motivation to change her dietary habits, I explained to Brett that storing fats *was not the only downside to eating the sugars and starches that provoke insulin responses. When those foods rapidly convert to sugar in the blood-stream, they can begin glycating the protein in body tissues, which is equivalent to the browning that causes food to discolor and toughen in storage. The sugar molecules attach themselves to collagen fibers, which in turn link to adjoining collagen molecules, causing the loss of skin elasticity and resulting in deep wrinkles.*

"That makes sense," Brett admitted. "But what do I do now? I've been eating this way for years—is it too late to stop the damage?" I explained that it is never too late to get started and emphasized that she think of this as a simple-to-follow, three-step program.

To focus on the glycation, I planned to start Brett on an anti-inflammatory supplement program that would include putting the power of peptides to work along with the dietary supplement carno-sine, a dipeptide (two amino acids) that has been shown to counter-act the effects of glycation. I also added benfotiamine, *a fat-soluble form of vitamin B$_1$ that has powerful anti-aging prop-erties (more about this threesome in chapter 7). I told Brett I would send her topical neuropeptide treatments to help with the wrinkles, fine lines, and loss of tone that were starting to manifest on her face and throat.*

First, however, Brett needed to be introduced to natural anti-oxidants. "I'm not going to give you a course in nutrition or bio-

chemistry," I said. "Instead you're going to base your food choices on the colors of the rainbow. Your sole criterion for food shopping is to choose deep, intense, and vibrantly colored foods. However," I warned, "Cheez Doodles do not count. This rule only applies to foods made by nature, not the laboratory."

Four weeks later, Brett dropped by my offices, radiating with vitality and health. Her skin appeared smooth and supple. I was delighted to notice that the bloom on her cheeks was natural. In fact, her business affiliation notwithstanding, Brett wore no makeup other than some light mascara and lip gloss.

"I can't tell you what a wonderful past month this has been," Brett confided. "I have always hated going to the supermarket—but by following your instructions, I discovered how much fun it could be. I consider my shopping trips as a little gift to my well-being. Each time, I challenge myself to find new rainbow foods to add to the growing list. I even started keeping a journal!"

Brett showed me the journal, which documented her first color-themed shopping trip. She had started in the produce aisle, where she selected a variety of baby greens, red cabbage, broccoli, string beans, red onions and even redder tomatoes, purple garlic, red and yellow bell peppers and a bright red chili pepper, alfalfa and broccoli sprouts, and a wide array of fresh herbs, including basil, parsley, thyme, rosemary, sage, oregano, and dill. Next stop, the fresh fruit aisles. Here Brett had selected the bluest blueberries, brilliant blackberries, and vivid red strawberries. Bright yellow lemons and vibrant orange cantaloupe, royal purple plums, a couple of deep red apples, and red-black bing cherries rounded out her selection. For condiments, Brett chose the rich green extra-virgin olive oil and an assortment of green and black olives. At the bulk foods department, Brett chose dark red kidney beans, black and red lentils, golden oats and barley, warm brown walnuts, almonds, and bright green pumpkin seeds. Final stop was the seafood department. Here Brett found rich red Alaskan sockeye salmon and Maine lobster, along with deep pink Alaskan king crab legs and shrimp.

"The best news is that even after four weeks, I feel like I have just begun to discover the abundant world of rainbow foods," Brett added. *"Each trip is like embarking on a new adventure. I believe I have undergone a total attitude adjustment regarding my food choices."*

Brett really had undergone an attitude transformation, and the benefits spilled over into many areas of her life. She had been casually dating Charles, a fellow executive, but when they began cooking and sharing meals together (a totally new experience for Brett), the relationship really began to take off. For the past two weekends, they had driven into the country in search of the freshest farmer's market fruits and vegetables. And they were planning a trip to an apple orchard in Vermont in the fall.

"You know, Dr. Perricone," Brett confessed, "before I started looking through that pair of rainbow-colored glasses you gave me, my life was essentially colorless. Now it is like a kaleidoscope of exciting new discoveries—every day. But what I find most amazing is how differently I look and feel!"

With any anti-aging, rejuvenation program, it is important to have at least a working knowledge of what works and why—just as it matters to understand why you need to avoid certain foods. In this chapter, aptly named Rainbow Foods, I discuss the science behind these antioxidant gifts from nature. As you will see, there is a huge abundance of benefits from these foods. My recommendation? To fulfill the Perricone Promise, enjoy as many of these foods as possible to obtain their full spectrum of age- and wrinkle-fighting properties.

Rainbow Foods: A Spectrum of Healthy Colors

At the beginning of this chapter, I said that plant pigments contain disease-preventive phytonutrients and anti-aging antioxidants. So what exactly are phytonutrients? Quite simply, *phyto* means "plant," therefore a phytonutrient is a nutrient derived from a plant. Most phytonutrients are powerful antioxidants, which, as we know, are nature's anti-inflammatory agents. And as *Time* magazine stated in February 2004, "The richer in color the better, since colorful plants tend to have the most antioxidants—good for mopping up free radicals produced during inflammation." It is both validating and encouraging to see mainstream media, such as *Time* magazine, acknowledge what I have long taught—that hidden inflammation is at the basis of many of the diseases associated with aging.

One of our best defenses against this hidden enemy is a diet rich in foods with anti-inflammatory phytonutrients: primarily colorful fruits and vegetables, as well as nuts, seeds, beans, and other legumes. It makes sense to eat as wide a variety of plant foods as possible, in order to achieve optimum phytonutrient protection against such avoidable degenerative conditions as heart disease, osteoporosis, arthritis, and wrinkled, sagging skin.

Researchers have identified almost two thousand different phytonutrient pigments in plant foods, many of which are antioxidants. In fact, researchers at the Agricultural Research Service's Human Nutrition Research Center on Aging at Tufts University in Boston developed a standardized test to measure the anti-oxidant potency of foods.

I expect that future research may tell us which foods exert the greatest preventive effect against free radicals, inflammation, and the disease conditions they promote. Until that time, the oxygen radical absorbance capacity (ORAC) scale identifies the most promising disease-preventive foods—at least in terms of antioxidant capacity. (Note that although raisins are second on the list, they, like all dried fruits, are very high in sugar and can cause an unwanted spike in blood sugar levels.)

It is recommended that we consume between 3,000 and 5,000 units a day. This isn't as much as it sounds—half a cup of blueberries, for instance, contains 2,400 units. The best idea is to eat both fruits and vegetables that add up to at least 5,000 ORAC units a day. And notice that these top twenty foods are among the most colorful in the rainbow spectrum.

COMPARING APPLES AND OREGANO

There are two key points to remember about various foods' ORAC scores. First, ORAC scores are designed to indicate the relative antioxidant capacity of edible substances within each category—an herb's antioxidant ranking among herbs tested, for instance, or a fruit or vegetable's antioxidant ranking among fruits and vegetables tested. And second, ounce for ounce, common culinary herbs possess greater antioxidant capacity than fruits or vegetables.

When you get to chapter 5, Spices of Life, you will notice that the ORAC scores for fruits and vegetables appear to be much higher than the ORAC scores for culinary herbs, when in fact culinary herbs have more antioxidant content and capacity per ounce. This is because different researchers use different, noncomparable measuring scales.

TOP TWENTY FOODS ON THE ORAC ANTIOXIDANT CAPACITY SCALE

ORAC units per 100 grams (about 3.5 ounces)

Fruits	ORAC Units	Vegetables	ORAC Units
Prunes	5,770	Kale	1,770
Raisins	2,830	Spinach	1,260
Blueberries	2,400	Brussels sprouts	980
Strawberries	1,540	Broccoli flowers	890
Raspberries	1,220	Beets	840
Plums	949	Red bell pepper	710
Oranges	750	Onion	450
Red grapes	739	Corn	400
Cherries	670	Eggplant	390
Kiwi fruit	602		
Pink grapefruit	483		

THE TOP OF THE RAINBOW

I urge you to read this chapter to gain a better understanding of the various phytonutrients, their benefits, and where they occur in foods. But to make it easy, here is a list of the most healthful rainbow foods.

- *Vegetables and herbs.* Alfalfa sprouts, bee pollen (dietary supplement), beet greens, bell peppers, broccoli, brussels sprouts, capers, cauliflower, chili peppers, chives, dark leafy greens (spinach, chard, collards, kale, mustard greens), dill, peppermint, red cabbage, tarragon, thyme, tomatoes.
- *Fruits.* Apples, apricots, berries (all types), cherries, kiwi fruit, pears, pomegranates, red grapes.
- *Beverages.* Black tea, green tea, pomegranate juice, red wine, white tea.

To help you identify (and thereby choose) the healthiest foods for skin and body maintenance, the rest of this chapter is divided into two parts. The first part concentrates on the phytonutrients—their categories, their names (some of which will be familiar, some won't), and their benefits. The second part is the Rainbow Chart. This chart divides foods by their predominant color and tells you which nutrients they contain.

Follow the Phytonutrients: Colorful Outside, Healthy Inside

As mentioned earlier, there are almost two thousand different phytonutrients that have so far been identified. In this chapter, I will concentrate on five of the most common—and healthful—categories:

1. Carotenoids
2. Limonoids and limonenes

3. Flavonoids
4. Flavon-3-ols
5. Glucosinolates and indoles

Don't be put off by the scientific names. All these phytonutrients are found in foods you are probably already eating. But my goal is to get you to eat *more* of these antioxidant, anti-inflammatory, peptide-boosting foods, and my guess is that when you know more about what they do for you, you'll be convinced that you should be adding them to your daily diet.

Consider the Carotenoids

Carotenoids (care-*ott*-en-oyds)—whose name derives from their role in giving carrots their color—are prominent among the pigments that color most fruits and vegetables. Carotenoids also lend their vivid yellow-orange-red hues to egg yolks and to wild Alaskan salmon, certain species of trout, shellfish, and birds such as the flamingo, all of which eat large quantities of carotenoid-rich foods. Carotenoids can be found in many green vegetables as well, but their color is masked by chlorophyll, a more predominant pigment.

Living things obtain their color, for the most part, from natural pigments. But the colors do more than just make them seem appealing; they also carry out a variety of important biological functions:

- Promote pro-vitamin-A activity, and are converted to retinol or vitamin A as needed.
- Reduce the risk of cardiovascular disease, probably because of their antioxidant, anti-inflammatory properties.
- Neutralize the free radicals responsible for general oxidative stress—the primary force behind inflammation.
- Reduce the risk of cancer, especially lung, bladder, breast, esophageal, and stomach cancers.
- Function as protective antioxidants in the retina (especially kale

and spinach), and may help prevent cataracts and macular degeneration.

- Block sunlight-induced inflammation in the skin, which leads to wrinkles and can cause skin cancer.
- Help reduce pain and inflammation.

The carotenoid family is divided into subgroups, two of which are known as carotenes and xanthophylls. For many years, beta-carotene attracted all the attention and was heavily studied. Recently, however, scientific interest has broadened, and other carotenoids are stimulating interest because of their potential health benefits. There is growing evidence that the way to get the most benefit is to consume a mix of carotenoids rather than large doses of any single one.

Here is the carotenoid family tree:

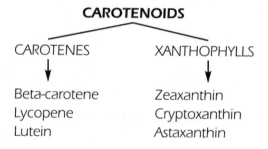

CAROTENES

Carotenes, which are found in apricots, bell peppers, chili peppers, tomatoes, parsley, beet greens, spinach, chard, collards, broccoli, kale, and romaine lettuce, enhance immune response, protect skin cells against UV radiation, and "spare" liver enzymes that neutralize carcinogens and other toxins. Remember, when eating any "sweet" carotene sources—such as carrots, winter squash, pumpkin, beets, or fruits, which all rank higher on the glycemic index—enjoy them in moderation and always eat some protein first.

- Beta-carotene is the familiar orange pigment and antioxidant included in many multivitamin supplements. The body can easily make beta-carotene into vitamin A, but it only converts as much as it needs, so it is considered a safer source of vitamin A, especially for pregnant women (excess vitamin A can harm the fetus).

- Lycopene is an antioxidant most abundant in tomatoes, but especially in processed tomato products. A diet rich in tomato juices, sauces, and soups appears to help prevent prostate, lung, stomach, and other cancers. Lycopene-rich foods may also help reduce the risk of cardiovascular disease by reducing LDL ("bad") cholesterol and lowering blood pressure.

- Lutein is found concentrated in dark, leafy greens (spinach, kale, collards, brussels sprouts), foods that appear to reduce the risk of cataracts and age-related macular degeneration. It migrates to the retina to protect photoreceptor cells from light-generated oxygen radicals. High levels of lutein in the blood correlate with a reduced risk of lung cancer.

XANTHOPHYLLS

Like carotenes, the xanthophyll (*zan*-tho-fill) group of carotenoids provides antioxidant protection. Xanthophylls also appear to protect vitamin A, vitamin E, and other carotenoids from oxidation. Among members of the xanthophyll family, three stand out for their antioxidant and preventive-health power: zeaxanthin, cryptoxanthin, and astaxanthin.

- Zeaxanthin, found in orange bell or chili peppers, collards, kale, spinach, lima beans, green beans, broccoli, brussels sprouts, cabbage, and lettuce, works with lutein to protect the eyes from sunlight damage.

- Cryptoxanthin, found in many of the same foods as zeaxanthin, may help prevent vaginal, uterine, and cervical cancers.

- Astaxanthin has been called "red gold from the sea" because it is the antioxidant champ of all carotenoids: ten times more potent than beta-carotene and one hundred times stronger than vitamin E. Pink and red sea creatures—such as wild Alaskan salmon, rainbow trout, shrimp, lobster, crawfish, and crabs—owe their beautiful coloring to astaxanthin in their diets. Wild Alaskan sockeye salmon is the astaxanthin champion, with a whopping 4.5 mg per four-ounce serving. In terms of antioxidant capacity, 4.5 mg of astaxanthin is equivalent to 450 mg of vitamin E—the amount widely recommended for optimum health.

Farm-raised Atlantic salmon has only one-quarter to one-half the astaxanthin of wild Alaskan salmon. Farmed fish that consume synthetic astaxanthin grow more slowly than fish that consume the same amount of astaxanthin from natural feed. This is an indication that synthetic astaxanthin does not function identically in salmon's bodies—and probably not in people's bodies, either.

WILD ALASKAN SALMON — THE KING OF THE SUPER FOODS

As my readers know, I've long urged people to eat wild salmon as frequently as possible, for many reasons, including:

1. Salmon is the heart-healthiest high-protein food of all.
2. Salmon is unique among protein foods in that it is powerfully anti-inflammatory. This is because salmon is by far the best source of long-chain omega-3 essential fatty acids (EPA, DHA, and others).
3. Salmon is the richest food source of a uniquely powerful antioxidant, anti-inflammatory orange pigment called astaxanthin, which you can read more about in this chapter.
4. Salmon is a rare dietary source of DMAE, the natural human neurochemical proven to help improve muscle tone in the face, thereby reducing wrinkles.

I always recommend wild-harvested Alaskan salmon, because it offers a far healthier fat profile than farmed

salmon, and contains only negligible amounts of the man-made pollutants (PCBs, pesticides) that occur at disturbingly high levels in typical farmed salmon. In addition, while the wild salmon fishery is universally declared safe and sustainable, salmon farms have created significant environmental problems that remain unresolved. So, I urge you to keep eating wild salmon as often as you can.

Pucker Up for Prevention: Limonoids and Limonenes

As their names suggest, these phytonutrients are found in sour citrus fruits such as lemons, limes, and grapefruit. While related to carotenoids, they do not provide color to foods, or as much antioxidant power—but limonoids and limonenes offer their own special benefits:

- Protect the lungs and alleviate chronic obstructive pulmonary disease.
- Help prevent cancer, by boosting the activity of detoxification enzymes in the liver.
- Lower blood cholesterol levels.
- Inhibit cancer in human breast cells and colon cancer in laboratory animals.

Favor the Flavonoids for Healthy Foods

Flavonoids (or bioflavonoids) offer many healthful properties. The term *flavonoid* generally includes all of the noncarotenoid antioxidants in vegetables and fruits.

Some foods rich in flavonoids include apples, bee pollen (a dietary supplement), broccoli, cabbage, capers, chili peppers, chives, cranberries, dill, elderberries, fennel, garlic, kale, leeks, lemons, onions, parsley, pears, peppermint, tarragon, and thyme.

Here's an overview of the beneficial properties of flavonoids:

- Fight free radicals, inflammation, and inflammatory conditions such as allergies.
- Help neutralize bacteria and viruses.
- Help protect against high blood pressure and sticky blood (platelet aggregation).
- Inhibit the growth of cancerous tumors.
- Protect the vascular system and strengthen the tiny capillaries that carry oxygen and essential nutrients to all cells.
- Help prevent cataracts.
- Support capillary strength and treat chronic venous insufficiency.

Most of the benefits of flavonoids stem from their antioxidant properties as powerful scavengers of free radicals. Another important property of flavonoids is their ability to raise the levels of glutathione, our primary antioxidant defense and an effective suppressor of chronic inflammation.

Flavonoids are also potent anti-inflammatory tonics, due to their effect on the cyclooxygenase (COX) enzymes. COX-1 enxymes help support healthy stomach, kidney, and blood platelet function, and protect the lining of the intestine. COX-2 enzymes, however, cause pain and inflammation.

One way to reduce active inflammation is to "inhibit" the COX enzymes. Aspirin, ibuprofen, and other nonsteroidal anti-inflammatory drugs (NSAIDs) inhibit both COX-1 and COX-2 enzymes. This is not good, since many of the COX-1 enzyme's effects are beneficial. The most common side effect of NSAIDs is a greater susceptibility to silent stomach bleeding, which helps to kill an estimated 100,000 Americans each year! Flavonoids have no such side effects, since they inhibit only the inflammatory COX-2 enzyme production.

COX-2 inhibitors are found in a variety of pain-relieving herbs, especially ginger and turmeric (as discussed in chapter 5). Common flavonoids called quercetin and myricetin, found in foods including capers, dill weed, fennel, buckwheat, bee pollen, onions, scallions, parsley, and rutabagas, are also powerful COX-2 inhibitors, in many cases working as well as prescription drugs.

Flock to Flavon-3-ols for Potent Protection

In 1535, sailors on French explorer Jacques Cartier's expedition to Canada fell seriously ill with scurvy. This degenerative disease of the connective tissues was caused by the typical seafarer's diet of the day—dried meat and biscuits. The crew was saved by the Native people's advice to drink tea made from the bark of a local pine tree.

In the 1930s, when the compound we now call vitamin C was identified as the elusive anti-scurvy nutrient in certain fruits and vegetables, it was named ascorbic (meaning "anti-scurvy") acid. But to scientists contemplating Cartier's rescue, the paltry vitamin C content of pine bark had always seemed insufficient to explain the rapid recovery of his scurvy-ridden crew. In fact, it was a class of antioxidants called flavon-3-ol polyphenols in pine bark tea—not its scarce vitamin C—that was primarily responsible for rescuing Cartier and his company.

It is the flavon-3-ol family that makes green tea so healthful. These compounds also make berries, pomegranates, apples, red wine, and grapes some of nature's top antioxidant foods.

Flavon-3-ols excel at four preventive-health tasks:

1. Protect against dangerous oxidation of LDL (bad) cholesterol—a key factor in the formation of plaque in the arteries.

2. Neutralize the free radicals responsible for general oxidative stress—the primary force behind inflammation.

3. Block the genetic and cellular damage that can lead to cancer, and inhibit the growth of tumors.

4. Block sunlight-induced aging of skin.

Here is the flavon-3-ol family tree:

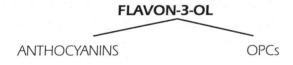

FLAVON-3-OL

ANTHOCYANINS   OPCs

ANTHOCYANINS

Anthocyanins are the antioxidant pigments that redden apples, berries, red-purple grapes (and therefore red wine), purple cabbage, eggplant—and autumn leaves. Elderberries and the Amazonian fruit called açaí are the richest anthocyanin sources by far. (See chapter 4, Ten Superfoods, for more about açaí—pronounced ah-sigh-*ee*—and where you can find the delicious açaí-based drink Sambazon.) Other rich sources, in rough order of anthocyanin content, include white tea, green tea, black tea, black currants, blueberries, blackberries, raspberries, cherries, strawberries, broad beans, red apples, apricots, red-purple cabbage, and buckwheat. Anthocyanins exhibit a variety of health benefits in animal and laboratory experiments:

- Protect against cancer by inhibiting inflammation, cancerous changes to cells, and tumor growth.
- Reduce premature brain aging and enhance memory.
- Help prevent macular degeneration, the leading cause of blindness in people over age sixty-five.
- Reduce oxidation of LDL cholesterol, reduce platelet aggregation (blood stickiness), dilate blood vessels, and improve overall heart function.
- Influence the body's hormone-like eicosanoids to reduce inflammation.

WHITE TEA: LESS CAFFEINE, MORE ANTIOXIDANTS

The term *white tea* refers to tea that has been minimally processed (air-dried and only slightly oxidized). Among all types of tea (green, oolong, black), white teas contain the highest levels of anthocyanins. White teas should be steeped in hot water—well shy of boiling, about 165 degrees Fahrenheit—for five to six minutes. This will ensure full flavor and a minimal caffeine yield of only 5 to 15 mg of caffeine per cup, versus 20 mg in green tea and 40 or 50 mg in black tea.

OPCS

OPCs (oligomeric proanthocyanidins) are concentrated in the seeds and outer coatings of many plants—which, unfortunately, are typically removed before eating. This explains why the best supplemental sources are grape seed extract, berry extracts, red wine extract, and pine bark extract (Pycnogenol). OPCs offer all of the benefits linked to anthocyanins, plus several additional and unique preventive-health and therapeutic attributes:

- Exert unsurpassed antioxidant effects in the body; they are eighteen times more effective than vitamin C, and fifty times more potent than vitamin E.
- Refresh the antioxidant capacity of vitamin C and vitamin E molecules exhausted by free-radical scavenging activities. This explains why some researchers call OPC "vitamin C_2."
- Are powerful anti-inflammatory agents.
- Promote healthy skin by preventing glycation (glycation = wrinkles).
- Help prevent cancer and can kill cancerous breast, lung, and gastric cells.
- Keep blood vessels strong: Since 1950, European doctors have prescribed pharmaceutical-grade OPC products to treat various conditions related to weak blood capillaries.
- May help prevent and treat urinary tract infections.
- Promote heart health.

GRAPES AND COCOA: PRO AND CON

Purple grape juice—a very rich source of flavon-3-ols—has up to three times the antioxidant capacity of orange, grapefruit, and tomato juices, which get their antioxidant power from carotenoids and flavonoids. One eight-ounce glass of Concord grape juice equals the antioxidant content of a full serving of rainbow fruits or vegetables. Grapes are also rich in a heart-healthy, anti-cancer antioxidant called resveratrol.

However, grape juice packs a high-glycemic—hence, inflammatory—punch that blunts much of its beneficial impact. You're better off getting your flavon-3-ols and resveratrol from supplements containing red wine extract or a traditional Chinese herb known as huzhang. Like grape juice and red wine, huzhang extract is very rich in flavon-3-ol antioxidants and resveratrol, and animal tests show that it protects skin very strongly against the sun's UV radiation. But unlike those beverages, huzhang extract is free of sugars and alcohol.

Cocoa powder is also extremely rich in flavon-3-ol antioxidants. In fact, cocoa contains double the flavon-3-ol antioxidants found in red wine, and five times as many as in green tea. While cocoa powder is virtually inedible until mixed with cocoa butter and/or sugar, you can enjoy its benefits in a reasonably healthful way by occasionally eating small amounts of very dark cocoa or chocolate, sweetened just enough to be palatable. Look for types that contain 70 percent or, even better, 85 percent cocoa solids—information you will find on the labels of most gourmet brands.

Super Antioxidants

One of the most exciting cancer-prevention breakthroughs was the discovery that cruciferous (croo-*sif*-er-us) vegetables such as broccoli, kale, brussels sprouts, cauliflower, and cabbage contain potent anti-cancer phytonutrients called indoles and glucosinolates. In fact, population studies indicate that *ounce for ounce, the cancer-protecting properties of cruciferous vegetables are greater than those of other fruits or vegetables, including foods with higher antioxidant levels.*

Three Colorful Standouts:
Pomegranates, Broccoli Sprouts, and Blueberries

There are three brightly colored foods that deserve special mention due to their superior antioxidant, anti-inflammatory, positive-peptide-boosting qualities. They are pomegranates, broccoli sprouts, and blueberries.

RED RIGHT FROM THE GARDEN OF EDEN: THE PREVENTIVE POWER OF POMEGRANATES

The pomegranate is one of the earliest cultivated fruits. Historical evidence suggests that humans first began planting pomegranate trees sometime between 4000 and 3000 BCE. Some historians believe that the apple made famous by Adam and Eve in the Garden of Eden was actually a pomegranate. Throughout history, this richly colored and delicious fruit has been revered as a symbol of health, fertility, and rebirth. In many medieval versions of the unicorn myth, the pomegranate tree to which it was bound represented eternal life, and some cultures also believed the fruit possessed profound and mystical healing powers. Today, science is proving that our forebearers may well have been on to something.

Pomegranate juice is a superior rainbow food, rich in flavon-3-ols. I always recommend eating the whole fruit or vegetable as opposed to drinking its juice, which usually lacks fiber and significant portions of the food's antioxidants. However, due to its extremely high antioxidant profile, drinking pomegranate juice made from the unsweetened extract is almost as good as eating the whole fruit—and you won't have to pick out this ancient delight's seemingly countless seeds!

GREEN MEANS GO FOR CANCER PREVENTION

Although they are not as widely known (or available), broccoli sprouts provide *even more* anti-cancer glucosinolates (ten to one hundred times more) and antioxidants by weight than mature broccoli. In addition, broccoli sprouts are especially rich in glucoraphanin—a substance that boosts the body's antioxidant defense systems. An animal study published in 2004 by the National Academy of Sciences showed that a diet including glucoraphanin-rich broccoli sprouts produced stronger antioxidant defenses, less inflammation, lower blood pressure, and better cardiovascular health in just fourteen weeks. Additional information is contained in the Sprouts section of chapter 4, Ten Superfoods.

THE BLUES FOR BETTER BALANCE AND BRAIN BOOSTING

The things we find out about certain foods are often quite surprising. Take the little blueberry, for instance. Who would think that this tiny fruit is one of the most beneficial rainbow foods you can find? It's true, though.

- Blueberries are brain food (it's not just fish anymore). Up until very recently, the belief has been that the decline in brain function, in both cognitive and motor aspects, is inevitable and irreversible. Consider the impaired sense of balance that is one of the telltale signs of aging. A young person can usually stand on one leg, even with eyes closed, much longer than an older person, who begins to sway and quickly needs to put down the raised leg in order to prevent a fall. We maintain our posture by automatically correcting against swaying motion; when the conduction of neural signals slows down with aging, we easily lose our balance. It turns out that daily doses of blueberries are the only treatment known that can reverse the deterioration of motor function with aging!
- The phytochemicals in the blueberry extract appear to speed up neural communication. Blueberry-supplemented neurons have a better ability to communicate with each other.

- Phytochemicals contained in blueberries prevent cell death and the loss of nerve growth factors.
- Blueberries allow the body a greater ability to release dopamine, an energizing, stimulatory neurotransmitter. Blueberries also protect us from the loss of dopamine cells that is normally seen with aging. By increasing brain energy production and maintaining youthful brain function, dopamine exerts an extremely important anti-aging effect. And, since dopamine decreases as we age, blueberries become even more important as we get older.

The Rainbow Chart: Your Colorful Guide to Healthy Eating

The following chart provides you with a rainbow of healthy choices that will give you radiant, glowing skin, help prevent degenerative diseases, and add years to your life.

Needless to say, not every rainbow food has been included. The chart is just a guideline to give you an idea of what kinds of food to include on your shopping list. The foods have been divided into color groups and then into their appropriate phytonutrient categories. Some foods are marked as "rich" in their particular phytonutrient; others contain the phytonutrient in lesser amounts; still others contain the phytonutrient, but are less desirable sources due to their high sugar content.

Next time you go to the grocery store or supermarket, make your cart the most colorful one there. You don't need to buy every color at once; try brightening up your menu a little at a time. And save some room for the Ten Superfoods in the next chapter—foods that add even more healthful benefits to your ever-expanding list of nutritious—and temptingly appetizing—meals.

	RED/ORANGE/YELLOW FOODS		
FOOD	HIGH IN	LESS ABUNDANT IN	LESS DESIRABLE SOURCE DUE TO HIGHER GLYCEMIC INDEX
Apple	Anthocyanins Flavonoids		
Apricot	Anthocyanins Beta-carotene		Zeaxanthin
Bee pollen	Flavonoids		
Beets			Carotene
Bell pepper	Beta-carotene Cryptoxanthin Zeaxanthin		
Cantaloupe		Beta-carotene Cryptoxanthin	
Carrots			Beta-carotene
Cherries	Anthocyanins		
Chili pepper	Beta-carotene Cryptoxanthin Flavonoids Zeaxanthin		
Corn			Lutein Zeaxanthin
Crabs	Anthocyanins		
Cranberries	Flavonoids		
Crawfish	Anthocyanins		
Garlic	Flavonoids		
Grapefruit	Limonoids		
Grape seed extract	OPCs		
Guava			Lycopene
Lemons	Limonoids		
Lobster	Anthocyanins		
Mango			Lutein Cryptoxanthin Zeaxanthin
Onion	Flavonoids		
Orange			Beta-carotene Cryptoxanthin Flavonoids

Food	High In	Less Abundant In	Less Desirable Source Due to Higher Glycemic Index
Orange			Limonoids Lutein Zeaxanthin
Papaya			Beta-carotene Cryptoxanthin Lutein Zeaxanthin
Peach			Beta-carotene Cryptoxanthin Lutein Zeaxanthin
Pear	Flavonoids		
Pomegranate	Anthocyanins		
Pumpkin			Lutein Zeaxanthin
Rainbow trout	Astaxanthin		
Raspberries	Anthocyanins		
Red cabbage	Anthocyanins		
Red grapes	OPCs		
Red wine	Anthocyanins		
Shrimp	Astaxanthin		
Strawberries	Anthocyanins		
Sweet potatoes			Anthocyanins Beta-carotene Lutein
Tangerine			Flavonoids
Tomato	Beta-carotene Lycopene		
Watermelon			Lycopene
Wild Alaskan salmon	Astaxanthin		
Winter squashes			Beta-carotene Cryptoxanthin Lutein Zeaxanthin
Yams			Anthocyanins Beta-carotene

GREEN FOODS			
FOOD	HIGH IN	LESS ABUNDANT IN	LESS DESIRABLE SOURCE OF
Apple	Flavonoids		
Beet greens	Beta-carotene		
Broad beans	Anthocyanins		
Broccoli	Cryptoxanthin Flavonoids Glucosinolate Lutein Zeaxanthin		
Broccoli sprouts	Glucosinolate		
Capers	Flavonoids		
Cauliflower	Glucosinolate		
Chard		Beta-carotene Lycopene	
Chives	Flavonoids		
Collard greens	Cryptoxanthin Zeaxanthin	Carotene	
Dill	Flavonoids		
Fennel	Flavonoids		
Green beans	Cryptoxanthin Lutein Zeaxanthin	Beta-carotene Lycopene	
Green cabbage	Cryptoxanthin Flavonoids Glucosinolate Lutein Zeaxanthin	Beta-carotene Lycopene	
Green tea	Anthocyanins		
Honeydew melon			Beta-carotene Lutein Zeaxanthin
Kale	Cryptoxanthin Flavonoids Glucosinolate Zeaxanthin	Carotene Lycopene	
Kiwi			Beta-carotene Lutein Zeaxanthin

Food	High In	Less Abundant In	Less Desirable Source Of
Leeks	Flavonoids		
Lettuce	Cryptoxanthin Lutein Zeaxanthin	Beta-carotene Lycopene	
Lima beans	Cryptoxanthin Lutein Zeaxanthin	Beta-Carotene Lycopene	
Lime	Limonoid		
Parsley	Beta-carotene Flavonoids		
Peas			Beta-carotene Lutein
Peppermint	Flavonoids		
Spinach	Cryptoxanthin Lutein Zeaxanthin	Beta-carotene Lycopene	
Tarragon	Flavonoids		
Thyme	Flavonoids		
Turnips			Glucosinolate

BLUE/PURPLE FOODS			
Food	High In	Less Abundant In	Less Desirable Source Of
Açaí	Anthocyanins		
Blackberries	Anthocyanins		
Black currants	Anthocyanins		
Black tea	Anthocyanins		
Blueberries	Anthocyanins		
Elderberries	Flavonoids		
Plums			Anthocyanins
Prunes			Beta-carotene Cryptoxanthin Lutein Zeaxanthin
Raisins			Anthocyanins

4 Ten Superfoods

Let food be thy medicine, thy medicine shall be thy food.
— HIPPOCRATES

Our lives are not in the lap of the gods, but in the lap of our cooks.
— LIN YUTANG, *THE IMPORTANCE OF LIVING*

NOW THAT YOUR SHOPPING CART IS FILLED with a rainbow of colorful, healthy foods, you're probably ready to start cooking. But wait. You might want to add a few more items before you finalize your menu plans. The purpose of adding the Ten Superfoods in this chapter to your diet is to enable you to construct a way of eating that will help you boost your peptide power to prevent inflammation and improve your immune system, to give you vibrant, glowing skin, and to enjoy extraordinarily good health.

Of course, there are more than just ten "superfoods." In fact, just about every brightly colored fruit and vegetable fits the category of a superfood, as do nuts, beans, seeds, and aromatic and brightly colored herbs and spices. The beneficial properties of each one of these superfoods could fill an entire book. The ten featured here were chosen because of their direct link to the Brain–Beauty Connection. These foods are rich in either the essential fatty acids (EFAs), antioxidants, or fiber, or—as in the case of açaí—all three! In addition, I have included foods that have been proven to lower or help regulate blood sugar levels—an extremely important factor for all of those concerned with slowing the aging process and preventing diabetes, obesity, wrinkles, and a host of degenerative diseases.

THE RIGHT FATS FOR FABULOUS SKIN

Although reducing the consumption of the wrong fats—particularly an excess of saturated fats, vegetable oils other than olive oil, and those fats known as trans-fatty acids—is a worthy goal, it's not healthy to try to eliminate all fat from your diet. In fact, this can be downright dangerous to your overall health, your brain power, and the condition of your skin. Fat is one of the nutrients your body requires, along with proteins, carbohydrates, and vitamins. The building blocks of fats and oils are called fatty acids. There exists a group of these fatty acids, known as essential fatty acids, which we can't make in our bodies. We must get them from the foods we eat. EFAs offer a variety of health benefits:

• Protect against heart disease.
• Protect against mental depression while preserving cognitive function.
• Lower blood pressure.
• Decrease the risk of blood clots.
• Lower the risk of colon, breast, and prostate cancers.
• Reduce inflammation, especially of autoimmune diseases.
• Keep skin supple and wrinkle-free.

Although many of these foods have reported medical benefits, remember at all times, that if you have any type of health problem or physical symptom, *do not self-diagnose or self-medicate*—even with a food or herb. Trust your medical professional first and foremost in this department. However, the ten foods included here do have incredible health benefits. Listed below are just some of the reasons to include these foods in your diet—every day:

• Prevent or reduce inflammation.
• Help regulate metabolism and burn body fat.

- Lower total cholesterol.
- Lower blood pressure.
- Help protect against heart disease.
- Help protect against cancer.
- Help protect organs from toxins.
- Promote digestive health.

Superfood Number 1:
Açaí, Nature's Energy Fruit

It may seem odd to start this list of superfoods with one you've likely never even heard of. But studies have shown that this little berry is one of the most nutritious and powerful foods in the world! Açaí (ah-sigh-*ee*) is the high-energy berry of a special Amazon palm tree. Harvested in the rain forests of Brazil, açaí tastes like a vibrant blend of berries and chocolate. Hidden within its royal purple pigment is the magic that makes it nature's perfect energy fruit. Açaí is packed full of antioxidants, amino acids, and essential fatty acids. Although açaí may not be available in your local supermarket, you can find it, often in juice form, in several health food and gourmet stores, such as Whole Foods and Wild Oats. A new product featuring the unsweetened pulp is now also available, and I highly recommend that you choose this form of açaí.

Açaí pulp contains:

- A remarkable concentration of antioxidants that help combat premature aging, with ten times more antioxidants than red grapes and ten to thirty times the anthocyanins of red wine.
- A synergy of monounsaturated (healthy) fats, dietary fiber, and phytosterols, to help promote cardiovascular system and digestive tract health.
- An almost perfect essential amino acid complex in conjunction with valuable trace minerals, vital to muscles.

FIGHT CHOLESTEROL WITH PHYTOSTEROLS

Phytosterols are plant compounds that are chemically similar to cholesterol. However, cholesterol, found in animal sources such as red meat, is absorbed easily when ingested and raises the body's own cholesterol levels. Phytosterols are difficult for the body to absorb, and (this is the good part) block cholesterol from being absorbed into the bloodstream. In other words, they actually help lower your cholesterol level. They also help prevent heart disease, help reduce inflammation in arthritis and other autoimmune diseases, and help control blood sugar levels in diabetes.

The fatty acid content in açaí resembles that of olive oil, and is rich in monounsaturated oleic acid. Oleic acid is important for a number of reasons. It helps omega-3 fish oils penetrate the cell membrane; together they help make cell membranes more supple. When the cell membrane is kept supple, all hormone, neurotransmitter, and insulin receptors function more efficiently. This is particularly important because high insulin levels create an inflammatory state, and, as you know, inflammation causes aging.

Superfood Number 2: The Allium Family

If açaí is the most exotic food on this list, the Allium family of foods is perhaps the most humble. Garlic, onions, leeks, scallions, shallots, and chives contain flavonoids that stimulate the production of glutathione—the tripeptide that is the liver's most potent antioxidant. Glutathione enhances elimination of toxins and carcinogens, putting the Allium family of vegetables at the top of the list for foods that can help prevent cancer. Here are just a few benefits from members of this family.

GARLIC

- Lowers total cholesterol (but raises HDL, or "good," cholesterol).
- Lessens the risk of atherosclerosis (hardening of the arteries).
- Lowers blood pressure.
- Reduces the risk of blood clots (which cause the *majority* of strokes and heart attacks).
- Destroys infection-causing viruses and bacteria.
- Reduces the risk of certain cancers, in particular stomach cancers.
- Produces more "natural killer" cells in the blood to fight tumors and infections.
- Helps fight against neurological diseases such as Alzheimer's.
- Enhances detoxification by reducing toxins.

For optimum effect, eat garlic raw. Cooking can destroy some of the allicin compound, which is the active constituent.

ONIONS

- Inhibit the growth of cancerous cells.
- Increase HDL cholesterol (especially when eaten raw).
- Reduce total cholesterol levels.
- Increase blood-clot-dissolving activity.
- Help prevent colds.
- Stimulate the immune system.
- Lower blood sugar levels in diabetes.
- Have anti-bacterial and anti-fungal properties.
- Reduce the risk of certain cancers.
- Help relieve stomach upset and other gastrointestinal disorders.

Onions contain two powerful antioxidants, sulfur and quercetin. Both help neutralize the free radicals in the body, and protect the membranes of the body's cells from damage.

LEEKS

Leeks have all of the healthy properties of the Allium family as described above. However, leeks also contain these nutrients:

- Vitamin B_6
- Vitamin C
- Folate
- Manganese
- Iron
- Fiber

This particular combination of nutrients makes leeks particularly helpful in stabilizing blood sugar, since they not only slow the absorption of sugars from the intestinal tract, but also help ensure that they are properly metabolized in the body. Remember, the stabilization of blood sugar is one of the most important goals of the Perricone Promise. Spikes in blood sugar accelerate aging, wrinkles, and a host of degenerative diseases.

We all know that onions and garlic are important for imparting delicious flavor to a meal. Adding leeks, however, elevates the flavor of the meal from delicious to sublime. They are particularly delicious with fish such as halibut, with chicken, and in fish and chicken soups.

Superfood Number 3: Barley

This ancient grain is sadly overlooked by today's culinary trendsetters. Yet it is one of the grains with the greatest health benefits, as well as delightful flavor and versatility. Barley can be used as a delicious breakfast cereal, in soups and stews, and as a rice substitute for dishes such as risotto.

Not only is barley a low-glycemic grain, but it is also high in both *soluble* and *insoluble fiber*. Soluble fiber helps the body metabolize fats, cholesterol, and carbohydrates, and lowers blood cholesterol levels. Insoluble fiber—commonly called roughage—promotes a healthy digestive tract and reduces the risk of cancers affecting it, such as colon cancer.

Dietary fiber is critical to health—yet few people in our modern society even come close to the recommended daily intake. Many experts believe that good health begins in the colon, and without sufficient fiber in the diet, we run the risk of a host of diseases ranging from hemorrhoids to colon cancer.

The fiber found in barley provides food for the beneficial bacteria in the large intestine. This is important because the "good" bacteria can crowd out the disease-causing bacteria in the intestinal tract, resulting in greater health and disease resistance.

Barley is sold in many forms, all of which are nutritious. But hulled barley, in which the outer hull (the bran) is left intact, is richer in fiber and contains more nutrients than other forms such as pearl barley or Scotch barley.

Eating hulled barley on a regular basis:

- Lowers blood cholesterol levels.
- Protects against cancer because the high fiber content helps speed food through the digestive tract, and because it is a good source of selenium, shown to significantly reduce the risk of colon cancer.
- Is a good source of niacin, the B vitamin that is cardio-protective.
- Slows starch digestion, which may help keep blood sugar levels stable.
- Provides high concentrations of tocotrienols, the "super" form of vitamin E.
- Provides lignans, phytochemicals that function as antioxidants. Women who consume lignans (also present in high levels in flaxseed) are less likely to develop breast cancer.

Superfood Number 4: Green Foods— Plant Power in Small Packages

When I talk about "green foods," I don't mean the ones in the green rainbow category of the last chapter. Here, I'm referring to a group of foods that includes young cereal grasses such as barley grass and wheat grass, as well as blue-green algae known as BGA. Nutritionally, they are close cousins to dark green leafy vegetables, but they offer far greater levels of nutrient density. In other words, an ounce of these concentrated green foods contains much more of the beneficial phytonutrients than is found in an ounce of green vegetables.

The results of many experimental studies show that green foods have marked beneficial effects on cholesterol, blood pressure, immune response, and cancer prevention. These effects are attributed in part to their high concentrations of chlorophyll.

Chlorophyll, the phytochemical that gives leaves, plants, and algae their green hues, is the plant equivalent of the oxygen-carrying red pigment hemoglobin in red blood cells. Dietary chlorophyll inhibits disease bacteria and exerts therapeutic effects on bad breath and internal odors.

WHEAT AND BARLEY GRASSES

Young cereal grasses—especially wheat and barley grass—are distinguished by their brilliant emerald-green hues. Before World War II, drugstores throughout the country—but especially in the Grain Belt states of the Midwest—sold tablets of dried wheat or barley grass as a kind of primitive vitamin supplement. Today, young wheat and barley grasses are dried and powdered to make dietary supplements, or picked fresh to process in juicing machines.

At the early grass stage of their growth, wheat and barley are closer to vegetables than grains in composition. This is important to note because while I strongly discourage eating wheat and wheat products, I believe wheat grass is an excellent addition to your diet.

The nutrient profiles of green cereal plants change quickly as they grow. In this process, the chlorophyll, protein, and vitamin content of cereal grasses declines sharply and the level of cellulose (indigestible fiber) increases. Over a period of several months, the green leafy cereal grasses become amber waves of grain bearing the kernels we harvest to make into flour—an unhealthy, pro-inflammatory food.

There is very little nutritional difference between wheat grass and barley grass, although it is important to note that barley grass acts as a free-radical scavenger that also reduces inflammation and pain, and wheat grass contains P4D1, a "gluco-protein" that acts like an antioxidant, reducing inflammation. It is also thought to help the body attack cancer cells.

You can get cereal grasses in powder or tablet form. Dried cereal grasses are certainly easier to handle than fresh, which must be juiced. However, fresh grass juice contains healthful enzymes not found in dried grass powder, and is likely to be higher in just about every phytonutrient found in cereal grass. Many juice bars and health-oriented markets offer these juices on their menus. You can check out the Resource Guide for suppliers of equipment and instructions to grow and "juice" your own wheat or barley grass.

BLUE-GREEN ALGAE (BGA): SPIRULINA, CHLORELLA, AND MORE

The single-celled plants known as blue-green algae (BGA) are sold in health food stores—and by multilevel marketing companies—as superior sources of protein, chlorophyll, carotenoid antioxidants, vitamins, minerals, and disease-preventive phytonutrients. There are several types of BGAs, the most popular being spirulina and chlorella.

The existing research, while lacking in many regards, suggests that BGAs exert some significant and perhaps unique preventive-health effects, most likely due to their polysaccharides, antioxidants, nucleic acids, and peptides.

Among other benefits, both spirulina and chlorella:

- Help diminish allergies such as hay fever.
- Help protect the liver from toxins.
- Reduce blood pressure and cholesterol.

- Help control symptoms of ulcerative colitis.
- Exert strong antioxidant and anti-inflammatory effects.

BGAs are rich in essential fatty acids, phenolic antioxidants, chlorophyll, B vitamins, carotenoids, and minerals such as calcium, iron, magnesium, manganese, potassium, and zinc. BGAs—especially spirulina—are also good sources of gamma linolenic acid (GLA), an omega-6 fatty acid with many healthful properties, which some people's bodies have trouble producing, and which is lacking in the standard American diet.

However, there are some cautionary notes about BGAs. They are often touted as rich sources of protein. In fact, dried BGA has relatively little protein, and you'd have to eat huge quantities—at great cost—to get a significant amount of protein. BGAs are also said to be rich in iron and carotenoids. That may be true, but it is far cheaper to get iron from food sources such as eggs, dark green leafy vegetables, or supplements, and you can get carotenoids more affordably from wild salmon and the colorful fruits and vegetables listed in chapter 3.

Extravagant claims are often made for the ability of dietary BGAs to provide energy and produce weight loss, without any substantial evidence for these assertions or logical reason to suppose that BGAs would suppress appetite as effectively as any number of fibrous plant foods. And since some kinds of blue-green algae (such as *Microcystis aeruginosa*) produce toxins called microcystins, which can cause liver damage and promote tumors, be sure that you buy only major national brands of BGA sold by very reputable retailers.

Superfood Number 5: Buckwheat—Seed, Grain, and Health Powerhouse

Though it is usually thought of as a grain, buckwheat is actually the seed of a broad-leafed plant related to rhubarb. While it is not a true grain, it is used like one in cooking, and it surpasses rice, wheat, and corn on almost every measure of healthfulness—including the fact that rice, wheat, and corn are high on the glycemic scale, thus provoking a quick spike in blood sugar levels, a proven promoter of systemic inflammation. Buckwheat, on the other hand, ranks low on the glycemic scale.

Hulled buckwheat kernels (called groats) are pale tan to green, while the roasted buckwheat groats known as kasha—a staple food in Eastern Europe—are dark brown with a nutty flavor. Kasha is often steamed in a stock with onions, olive oil, and fresh parsley, and you can combine equal parts plain buckwheat groats and oats, and cook the mix to enjoy as a hot breakfast cereal topped with berries. Buckwheat has been cultivated for at least a thousand years in China, Korea, and Japan, where it is often enjoyed in the form of soba noodles—a form that's become increasingly popular in the West as a healthy substitute for wheat pasta.

Buckwheat has more protein than rice, wheat, millet, or corn, and is high in the essential amino acids lysine and arginine, in which major cereal crops are deficient. Its unique amino acid profile gives buckwheat the power to boost the protein value of beans and cereal grains eaten the same day. Yet buckwheat contains no gluten—the source of protein in true grains—and is therefore safe for people with gluten allergy or celiac disease.

In addition, buckwheat protein offers unique health-promoting properties:

- Buckwheat is the unsurpassed cholesterol-lowering food studied to date.
- It helps reduce and stabilize blood sugar levels following meals—a key factor in preventing diabetes and obesity.
- Like the widely prescribed ACE inhibitor hypertension drugs, buckwheat proteins reduce the activity of angiotensin converting enzyme (ACE), thereby reducing hypertension.

WHY BUCKWHEAT IS BETTER THAN GRAINS

- *More vitamins and minerals.* Compared with true grains, buckwheat is high in minerals, especially zinc, copper, and manganese (13 to 89 percent of their recommended dietary allowances).

- *Healthier fat profile.* Unlike true grains, buckwheat's low fat content is skewed toward monounsaturated fatty acids—the type that makes olive oil so heart-healthful.
- *Healthier starch and fiber profile.* The fiber in true grains (other than barley) is largely insoluble, while a considerable portion of buckwheat's dietary fiber is the soluble type that makes oats so heart-healthful, and helps reduce blood cholesterol levels and the risk of colon cancer. In addition, buckwheat is high in resistant starch, which also enhances colon health, and serves to reduce blood sugar levels.
- *Reduces high blood pressure and LDL (bad) cholesterol,* and discourages obesity. Most recently, a buckwheat extract was found to substantially reduce blood glucose levels in diabetic rats—a promising finding that should lead to similar research in human diabetics. This blood sugar benefit is attributed in part to rare carbohydrate compounds called fagopyritols (especially D-chiro-inositol), of which buckwheat is by far the *richest food source* yet discovered.
- *Contains flavonoids for heart and circulatory health.* In addition to its marked nutritional benefits, buckwheat has been traditionally prized as a "blood-building" food. Modern science attributes this ancient reputation to buckwheat's high levels of antioxidant polyphenols—especially rutin (a bioflavonoid), which supports the circulatory system and helps prevent recurrent bleeding caused by weakened blood vessels, as in hemorrhoids and varicose veins. Finally, rutin acts as an ACE inhibitor, and contributes to buckwheat's ability to reduce high blood pressure.

Superfood Number 6: Beans and Lentils

There are good reasons that beans occupy two places on the U.S. Department of Agriculture's Food Guide Pyramid. The first is alongside high-protein foods such as meat, eggs, poultry, and fish, and the second is among vitamin-rich vegetables. The beneficial phytochemicals found in beans offer other preventive health attributes not reflected in the USDA's pyramid. The multifaceted nutrition and prevention powers of beans—a category that encompasses common beans (kidney, black, navy, pinto), chickpeas (garbanzo beans), soybeans, dried peas, and lentils—make them an anti-aging dietary necessity.

Beans are low in fat (except for soybeans), calories, and sodium, but high in complex carbohydrates and dietary fiber, and they offer modest amounts of essential fatty acids—mostly omega-6s (only soybeans have significant amounts of omega-3 fatty acids). They are also an excellent source of protein, needing only to be combined with grains such as barley or oats to provide all the amino acids necessary to make a complete protein for vegetarians who do not have other sources of protein for their meals.

Beans are extremely beneficial in an anti-diabetes diet because they rank low on the glycemic scale, which means that they do not cause the inflammatory, hunger-inducing spike in blood sugar levels associated with refined grains and baked goods. Beans offer ample fiber: One cup of cooked beans can provide as much as 15 grams of dietary fiber—more than half the recommended daily value of 25 grams—and this fiber is released into the bloodstream slowly, providing energy and satiation for a sustained period. However, I recommend no more than a quarter to a half cup of cooked beans per meal.

Dry beans and lentils are a staple of many cuisines worldwide. They have been one of the most nutritious foods available for thousands of years, and continue to be so. In addition, beans and lentils are extremely versatile. They can be combined with fragrant herbs and vegetables and made into delicious soups. They can be used in salads, or pureed and served as a dip or spread. Chickpeas and lentils can also be ground into a high-protein, low-glycemic flour.

HEALTHY BENEFITS OF BEANS

Beans are heart-healthy for a number of reasons in addition to their fiber content:

- They are a good source of potassium, which may help reduce your risk of high blood pressure and stroke. More than 80 percent of American adults do not consume the daily value for potassium (3,500 mg), and just half a cup of cooked dry beans contains as much as 480 mg, with no more than 5 mg of sodium.
- Dry beans are a good source of folic acid, which protects against heart disease by breaking down an amino acid called homocysteine. (One cup of cooked dry beans provides about 264 mcg of folate, or more than half the recommended daily intake of 400 mcg.) High levels of homocysteine in the blood, or inadequate amounts of dietary folate, can triple the risk of heart attack and stroke. Folate is also key in preventing birth defects, and may help reduce the risk of several types of cancer because it plays an important role in healthy cell division and is crucial to the repair of damaged cells.
- In a study of almost ten thousand men and women, those who ate beans four or more times a week cut their risk of coronary heart disease by about 20 percent, compared with those who ate beans less than once a week. It appears that this health benefit was independent of other health habits, since adjustments to account for other important cardiovascular disease risk factors produced minimal change in the risk estimates.
- Other studies show that within two to three weeks, diets high in either canned or dry beans (three to four ounces per day) reduce blood cholesterol levels by 10 percent or more—an effect that can result in a 20 percent decrease in the risk of coronary heart disease.
- Beans and lentils have the same potent anti-inflammatory antioxidants—flavonoids and flavonals—found in tea, fruits, grapes, red wine, and cocoa beans. In particular, the reddish flavonal pigments in bean and lentil seed coats exert antioxidant activity fifty times greater than vitamin E, protect against oxidative damage to cell membrane lipids, promote healthy collagen and cartilage, and restore the antioxidant powers of vitamins C and E after they've battled free radicals.

- Beans are among the richest food sources of saponins, chemicals that help prevent undesirable genetic mutations.

PREPARING BEANS

Generally speaking, the larger the beans, the longer they need to soak; and the longer you soak beans, the faster they cook. Dry chickpeas, beans, and whole dry peas need about eight hours of soaking.

If you forget to soak them the night before, just do it before you leave in the morning and they'll be ready to cook when you get home. Or add three times as much water as you have beans, bring them to a boil for a few minutes, remove from the heat, and let sit for an hour. Throw out the soaking water and cook as usual. You can also use a pressure cooker, which will reduce the cooking time by more than half, and reduce nutrient loss. (Of course, you can just drain and rinse canned beans, and add them directly to salads, soups, or curries.) You can also prepare large batches to freeze in meal-sized portions—cooked beans freeze well.

Well-soaked beans take forty-five minutes to an hour to cook, depending on the variety. Cook beans until soft, and then rinse them thoroughly, because the residual starch on the surface feeds the harmless bacteria in your gut, which then release gas. Some of the gas-producing starch stays in the soaking water, so don't cook with it.

You can prevent gas by adding beans to your diet gradually, eating just a bite or two per day to start until your body adjusts. Drinking ample fluids also helps. You can also try an enzyme supplement such as Beano, sold in most supermarkets, which will digest the gas-producing sugars. Just put a few drops on the first bite of food.

PREPARING LENTILS

Like other legumes, lentils are low in fat and high in protein and fiber, but they have the added advantage of cooking quickly. Lentils do not need presoaking. Simply remove any debris, then rinse and boil them. Red lentils take only twenty minutes, green lentils take thirty to forty-five minutes, and brown lentils cook in forty-five to sixty minutes. Do not add salt to the cooking lentils, because this can toughen them. Like beans, lentils will keep almost indefinitely in a cool, dry place. Their colors may fade slightly after long storage, but their flavor and nutrition won't. Lentils are the perfect way to add protein, fiber, and all the antioxidant benefits of this food group to any meal. And they taste wonderful, adapting themselves to a wide range of aromatic spices and herbs—particularly turmeric and ginger.

Superfood Number 7: Hot Peppers

The term *peppers* encompasses a diverse group of plants, ranging from the popular sweet green or red bell pepper to the fiery hot habanero or even more lethal Scotch bonnet. When Columbus tasted the small, hot red "berries" he found on his Caribbean voyages, he believed he had reached India—where Europeans obtained black pepper—and called them red pepper. In truth, the Native peoples of the Americas had been growing and enjoying sweet and chili peppers for an estimated seven thousand years. Soon after Columbus's ships brought them back to Spain, traders spread them around the world, transforming cuisines—and people's preventive-health prospects—from Morocco to Hungary, and India to China.

Peppers—whether sweet bell or hot chili—are members of the plant genus *Capsicum* (*cap*-sih-kum), a term that comes from the Greek word *kapto*, which means "to bite."

All peppers contain compounds called capsaicinoids. This is especially true of chili peppers, which derive their spicy heat—as well as extraordinary anti-inflammatory, analgesic, anti-cancer, heart-healthy effects—from very high levels of capsaicinoids, the most common form of which is capsaicin.

In addition to capsaicin, chilies are high in antioxidant carotenes and flavonoids, and contain about twice the amount of vitamin C found in citrus fruits. Almost any dish, from homemade soups, stews, and chili to stir-fries, salads, and salsas, can benefit from small amounts of hot peppers.

CAPSAICIN'S HEALTH BENEFITS

- *Headache help.* As you learned in chapter 2, Substance P is the key transmitter of pain to the brain. In fact, Substance P is the body's main mechanism for producing swelling and pain throughout the trigeminal nerve, which runs through the head, temple, and sinus cavity. When the nerve fibers come in contact with Substance P, they react by swelling—an effect that yields headaches and sinus symptoms. Research has shown that eating foods that contain capsaicin can suppress Substance P production. Clinical studies have shown that capsaicin is extremely effective for relieving and preventing cluster headaches, migraine headaches, and sinus headaches.
- *Arthritis relief.* People suffering from arthritis pain typically have elevated levels of Substance P in their blood and in the synovial fluid that bathes their joints. Again, eating capsaicin foods—or applying a topical cream that contains capsaicin—can offer relief.
- *Capsaicin as spicy sinus soother.* Capsaicin also possesses powerful anti-bacterial properties, and is very effective in fighting and preventing chronic sinus infections (sinusitis). This purely natural chemical will also clear out congested nasal passages like nothing else, and is helpful in treating sinus-related allergy symptoms. Small daily doses of capsaicin have even been shown to prevent chronic nasal congestion.

- *Capsaicin as anti-inflammatory.* In recent years, researchers have discovered that capsaicin is a potent anti-inflammatory, and have even pinpointed how it works to fight chronic inflammation. The nuclei of human cells contain chemicals called nuclear transcription factors (NTFs), two of which—activator protein 1 (AP-1) and NF-kappa B—are especially important targets when it comes to prevention of cancer and premature aging of skin. Each of these NTFs can be "activated" by ultraviolet light and free radicals, producing a pro-inflammatory chain reaction that promotes premature aging and a wide variety of degenerative diseases. The antioxidant alpha lipoic acid (ALA) is extraordinarily efficient at keeping these two key NTFs from kicking off a pro-inflammatory cascade reaction. (This is why I use ALA extensively in my topical treatments and recommend it as a dietary supplement.) And as it turns out, nature offers several other effective NTF-activation blockers, including the capsaicin in chilies and the yellow pigment curcumin in turmeric.

- *Gastric relief.* A recent study on gastric disorders at Duke University showed that capsaicin may actually lead to a cure for certain intestinal diseases. The Duke team found that a specific nerve cell receptor appears to be necessary to initiate the development of inflammatory bowel disease (IBD), a general term given to a variety of chronic disorders in which the intestine becomes inflamed, resulting in recurring abdominal cramps, pain, and diarrhea. The cause of IBD is unknown, and it is believed that up to two million Americans suffer from this disorder.

- *Capsaicin versus cancer.* Several recent studies have shown that capsaicin may actually prevent the growth of certain types of cancer. In particular, several clinical studies conducted in Japan and China showed natural capsaicin directly inhibits the growth of leukemic cells. Although these studies used pure capsaicin directly injected into isolated diseased cells in a laboratory setting, scientists have also concluded that daily consumption of hot peppers (thus capsaicin) may prevent certain types of cancer. Throughout South America, intestinal, stomach, and colon cancer rates are very low compared to those in the United States. It is widely regarded by medical experts that this low cancer rate may be tied to the large amounts of capsaicin in Latin Americans' diets, since nearly every main dish in their normal diet contains some form of capsaicin-based food, particularly hot cayenne and jalapeño peppers. Of course, we must also take into consideration the fact that these cultures consume fiber-rich beans on a daily basis.

- *Capsaicin as fat burner.* Capsaicin is an active ingredient in many of the most popular "fat-burning" supplements on the market. A thermogenic agent, capsaicin helps increase overall metabolic activity, thus helping the body burn calories and fat. Since the Food and Drug Administration (FDA) banned the herb ephedra, supplement manufacturers have been searching for new thermogenic ingredients, and many have added chilies to the mix. While capsaicin replaces some of ephedra's metabolic effects, it doesn't have that herb's negative, stimulant effects on heart rate. In fact, capsaicin is an actively heart-healthy supplement.

THE SCOVILLE SCALE:
HOT, HOTTER, HOTTEST

Capsaicin is mainly found in hot pepper plants from the *Capsicum* genus. While most varieties are found in South America, where chilies originated, there are also capsicum varieties in Africa, India, and even China. Like bell peppers, which also belong to the capsicum family, not all chili peppers are hot. For example, paprika is from the capsicum family, but it's mild at best. On the other hand, paprika's cousin cayenne is scorching hot. It all depends on the heat factor within a particular plant.

Hot peppers even have their own heat measurement scale, known as Scoville Units. Mostly used in the food industry, the Scoville heat scale is regarded as the most accurate way to measure the true hotness of a pepper plant. Developed in 1912 by botanist Wilbur Scoville, a pepper's Scoville Unit number is based on how much the ground chili needs to be diluted before no heat is detected. Scoville Units measure the perception of heat in multiples of 100, with bell peppers setting the heat-free baseline at 0 Scoville Units, pure capsaicin measuring more than 16 million Scoville Units, and most popular types ranking around 30,000 Scoville Units. Until recently, habanero peppers held the world record, with some varieties scoring a searing 300,000 Scoville Units. In 2000, however, Indian research scientists tested a chili pepper called Naga Jolokia from the remote northeastern province of Assam. This devilishly hot Indian chili now holds the dubious distinction of being the world's hottest, with a reported score of 855,000 Scoville units.

About 80 percent of a chili's capsaicin is found in the ribs and seeds, which can be removed to reduce its heat. Capsaicin is also distributed unevenly, in much smaller amounts, throughout the flesh of a chili pepper.

Aerosolized capsaicin, better known as pepper spray (often used to fend off potential attackers), is now being used to fend off sinus infections, allergies, and headaches, thanks to a new nasal spray packed with hot pepper extract. To learn more, visit the Resource Guide at the back of this book.

Always exercise a great deal of care when preparing hot peppers, to avoid injury. Check at the produce department to select the pepper with the right degree of heat for your palate. Use rubber gloves when chopping and seeding, and don't touch your eyes during preparation: The oil in the hot peppers will cause a burning sensation—advice spoken with the voice of painful experience!

Superfood Number 8: Nuts and Seeds

If you want to dramatically decrease your risk of cancer, heart disease, and diabetes, control your weight with no hunger pangs, and reduce the visible signs of aging such as wrinkles and sagging skin, I recommend that you "go nuts."

Here's how:

- When thoughts turn to food between meals, enjoy a handful of raw, unsalted nuts. They're extremely filling and satisfying—and healthful.
- Add some nuts to regular meals—a tablespoon of chopped almonds on your oatmeal, a tablespoon of walnuts in your lunchtime salad, or a Hazelnut-Encrusted Wild Salmon Fillet (see the recipe in appendix A). Nuts are so versatile, they can take the place of flour and bread crumbs—with a lot more flavor and health benefits. Just remember, as with all things, to use moderation.

NUTS, SEEDS, AND HEART HEALTH

Studies involving more than 220,000 people show that "nutty" diets help reduce the risk of heart disease, the leading killer of both men and women in the United States. This should come as no surprise: Nuts contain powerful antioxidants and anti–inflammatories, and, like so many other diseases, heart disease is an inflammatory condition.

For example, consider these findings:

- The famous Seventh Day Adventists Study followed more than thirty thousand church members over a twelve-year period. The results showed that even in this healthy-living, largely vegetarian group, those who ate nuts at least five times per week cut their risk of dying from coronary heart disease (CHD) by 48 percent, compared with those who ate nuts less than once weekly. They also cut their risk of a nonfatal heart attack by 51 percent.

- In a study involving more than three thousand African American men and women, those who consumed nuts at least five times a week cut their risk of dying from CHD by 44 percent, compared with those who ate nuts less than once weekly.
- The results of the fourteen-year-long Nurses' Health Study—which involved more than eighty-six thousand women—indicate that women who consume more than five ounces of nuts weekly will cut their risk of CHD by 35 percent, compared with those who eat less than one ounce per month. (Similar reductions were seen in the risk of death from CHD and nonfatal heart attacks.) And the seventeen-year Physicians' Health Study involving more than twenty-one thousand men found that those who consumed nuts at least twice a week cut their risk of sudden cardiac death by 53 percent, compared with those who rarely ate nuts. (There was no significant decrease in the risk of nonfatal heart attack or nonsudden CHD death.)

Nuts enhance heart health because of their unique protein, fat, sterol, and vitamin profile:

- *Heart-healthy protein.* Most nuts are high in arginine, an amino acid that reduces cholesterol levels and, as a precursor to nitric oxide, dilates blood vessels, thus reducing blood pressure and the risk of angina, congestive heart failure, and heart attack.
- *Heart-healthy fats.* Most of the fat in nuts consists of the polyunsaturated omega-3 and omega-6 varieties that reduce blood cholesterol levels. Numerous clinical studies have found that almonds, hazelnuts, macadamia nuts, peanuts, pecans, pistachio nuts, and walnuts all reduce total cholesterol and LDL cholesterol in people with normal-to-high cholesterol levels. And the fatty compounds in nuts' phytosterols inhibit accumulation of fats in artery walls, which promotes angina, strokes, and heart attacks.
- *Heart-healthy vitamins.* Vitamin E—an antioxidant in which almonds are especially rich—helps prevent the oxidation of cholesterol that leads to fatty buildup in the arteries. The B

vitamin folate, found in many nuts, lowers high blood levels of homocysteine, a strong predictor of heart disease.

- *Heart-healthy minerals.* Nuts and seeds are generally rich in calcium, magnesium, and potassium, all of which serve to reduce blood pressure.
- *Heart-healthy phytochemicals.* The coatings of all nuts and seeds—such as the thin brown papery layer coating almonds and peanuts—are rich in the antioxidant polyphenols associated with reduced risk of heart disease. (Processed nuts and seeds possess fewer of these antioxidants; choose raw nuts in the shell when possible.) Walnuts in particular are high in alpha linolenic acid, an essential fatty acid that is protective to the heart and circulation.

NUTTY, SEEDY CANCER FOES

The particular fats, antioxidant polyphenols, and proteins that make nuts heart-healthy also help prevent cancer:

- Phytic acid is a natural plant antioxidant found in nuts and seeds. It serves as a potent antioxidant to help preserve seeds, and may reduce the rate of colon cancer and other inflammatory bowel diseases via the same mechanism.
- The coatings of all nuts and seeds are rich in the antioxidant polyphenols associated with reduced risk of cancer. (This is another reason to choose raw nuts and seeds in the shell, versus processed nuts and seeds.)
- Beta-sitosterol and campesterol—two of the phytosterols found in most nuts—appear to suppress breast and prostate tumors.
- The amino acid arginine, which is abundant in most nuts—especially almonds—also inhibits tumor growth and boosts immunity.
- Walnuts are especially helpful because they contain ellagic acid—the cancer-fighting polyphenol antioxidant also found in pomegranates and red raspberries.
- Selenium, another key antioxidant factor and cancer-preventive mineral, is particularly abundant in Brazil nuts.

IN A NUTSHELL: A RICH BUT SLIMMING SNACK

While it may seem odd, diets that include moderate amounts of nuts—which are inherently high in fat and calories—help prevent obesity and even reduce weight. One study found that dieters on a calorie-controlled, moderate-fat (35 percent of calories) plan that included nuts and other good fats lost as much weight as dieters on a 20-percent-fat calorie-controlled plan. The moderate-fat group also maintained their weight loss better than the low-fat group over the eighteen-month test period and beyond—likely because the "moderate-fat, nuts-allowed" group reported fewer problems with sensations of hunger than the low-fat diet group did.

BUYING AND STORING NUTS

The appetite-suppressing and health benefits of nuts and seeds are lost when they are salted, oiled, roasted, stale, or rancid. And the fats in nuts and seeds are susceptible to oxidation after they are shelled and exposed to light and air—a process that destroys their nutritional value and degrades their taste.

Accordingly, nuts and seeds should be bought in small quantities and stored in their shells—which shield them against oxidation—in a cool, dry place. Discard any shells with cracks, as well as any nuts or seeds that are discolored, limp, rubbery, moldy, or shriveled, or that have an "off" smell or taste. Store any shelled nuts or seeds in an airtight container in your refrigerator (one week or less) or freezer. Last, prepare your own crushed or slivered nuts, to ensure maximum freshness.

The enzyme inhibitors and phytates in nuts limit the availability of their nutrients. To maximize the nutritional value of nuts, soak them in salted water for six to eight hours, drain out the water, and oven-dry the nuts on a cookie sheet on low heat.

NUTS AND SEEDS IN YOUR DIET

Nuts and seeds add texture and flavor to salads and many recipes. Of course, they also make great snacks. Many people like to snack on nut butters, spread on crackers or fruit. I do not recommend buying nut butters prepared on site in stores, because you can't know whether the grinder is clean, and because the fresh nut butter is exposed to air and light as it emerges from the grinder. Frankly, you are better off buying premade nut butters from reputable natural food brands that do not add hydrogenated oils. It is fairly easy to make your own nut and seed butters in a food processor: Just add oil as needed. As with nuts and seeds, keep homemade nut butters and open, store-bought nut butters in airtight containers in the refrigerator.

I recommend eating one serving of nuts or seeds (a quarter cup) every day. And, in addition to olive oil, it is healthy to cook with macadamia, peanut, sesame, or canola oil instead of butter, margarine, or shortening. Needless to say, you need to consider the distinct flavor of each nut oil: Peanut oil is ideal for many Asian meals. Never cook with fragile flax, hemp, or walnut oils, because their delicate omega-3 fatty acids will oxidize under the exposure to heat and air and light. Use flaxseed, walnut, hemp seed, or olive oil in homemade salad dressings. Whenever possible, buy organic nuts, seeds, and oils. All nuts and seeds are healthful in moderation: The key is to eat a variety. However, certain ones stand out for their exceptionally healthful fatty acid composition. I recommend the following nuts and seeds because they are the highest in either omega-3 or omega-9 (monounsaturated) fatty acids. Both fatty acids are heart-healthy; omega-3s are powerful anti-inflammatory agents as well. The fatty acid content of each nut or seed is expressed here as a percent of its total fat content. (*Note:* The percentage figures provided are averages, as the fatty acid content of nuts and seeds varies considerably among data sources.)

- *Highest in omega-9 monounsaturated fatty acids.* Macadamia (50 percent), pecans (45 percent), almonds (42 percent), filberts (38 percent), pistachios (35 percent), Brazil nuts (32 percent), peanuts (23 percent), sesame seeds (21 percent). *Note:* Unlike most nuts, pistachios are high in antioxidant carotenoids.

- *Highest in omega-3 polyunsaturated fatty acids.* Flaxseed (50 percent), walnuts (8 percent), pumpkin seeds (7 percent).

Superfood Number 9: Sprouts

Sprouts are a highly nutritious food. Grown locally year-round, sprouts are a good source of protein and vitamin C. In the interest of providing the finest nutritional information regarding sprouts, their history, nutrition, and variety of uses, I contacted the International Sprout Growers Association (ISGA), which graciously granted me permission to share much of their scientific and historical information in this book.

The ISGA was founded in 1989 as a nonprofit organization to promote the sprout industry and to encourage the exchange of information among sprout growers and commercial suppliers. Visit them at www.isga-sprouts.org for more information as well as some outstanding recipes.

WHAT IS A SPROUT?

A sprout is produced when a seed starts growing into a vegetable. Sprouts can grow from the seeds of vegetables, grains, legumes, buckwheat, and beans. Sprouts vary in texture and taste. Some are spicy (radish and onion sprouts), some are hardy and often used in Asian cuisines (mung bean), while others are more delicate (alfalfa), adding texture and moistness to salads and sandwiches.

WHY SPROUTS?

There are a great many reasons to eat sprouts. As we age, our body's ability to produce enzymes declines. Sprouts are a concentrated source of the living enzymes and "life force" that is lost when foods are cooked or not picked fresh from your own garden. Additionally, due to their high enzyme content, sprouts are also much easier to digest than the seed or bean from which they came. Sprouts are such a nutrition power-house, they even have their own superhero—"Sproutman," aka Steve Meyerowitz (www.sproutman.com). The following information from Sproutman provides a comprehensive answer to the question *Why should I eat sprouts—aren't fresh vegetables and fruit enough?*

> The National Cancer Institute and the National Institutes of Health both recommend eating 5 fresh fruits and vegetables every day. A great way to help reach that goal is to include sprouts. Alfalfa sprouts have more chlorophyll than spinach, kale, cabbage or parsley. Alfalfa, sunflower, clover and radish sprouts are all 4 percent protein. Compare that to spinach at 3 percent, Romaine lettuce at 1.5 percent, Iceberg lettuce at 0.8 percent, and even milk at only 3.3 percent. . . . Meat is 19 percent and eggs are 13 percent protein (but 11 percent fat). . . . Soybean sprouts have twice the protein of eggs and only $\frac{1}{10}$ of the fat. . . . Radish sprouts have 29 times more Vitamin C than milk (29 mg vs. 1 mg) and 4 times the Vitamin A (391 IU vs. 126).
>
> Alfalfa, radish, broccoli, clover and soybean contain concen-trated amounts of phytochemicals (plant compounds) that can protect us against disease. Canavanine, an amino acid analog present in alfalfa, demonstrates resistance to pancreatic, colon and leukemia cancers. Plant estrogens in these sprouts function similarly to human estrogen but without the side effects. They increase bone formation and density and prevent bone break-down (osteoporosis). They are helpful in controlling hot flashes, menopause, PMS and fibrocystic breast tumors. And, in addition to higher levels of glucosinolates and isothiocyanates, broccoli sprouts are especially rich in glucoraphanin—a substance that boosts the body's antioxidant defense systems. A study pub-lished in 2004 by the National Academy of Sciences showed that a diet including glucoraphanin-rich broccoli sprouts pro-duced stronger antioxidant defenses, less inflammation, lower blood pressure and better cardiovascular health in just 14 weeks.
>
> Alfalfa sprouts are one of our finest food sources of saponins, which lower the bad cholesterol and fat but not the good HDL

fats. . . . Saponins also stimulate the immune system by increasing the activity of natural killer cells such as T-lymphocytes and interferon. . . . Sprouts also contain an abundance of highly active antioxidants that prevent DNA destruction and protect us from the ongoing effects of aging.

As a physician whose field has long been anti-aging, I strongly believe that Steve "Sproutman" Meyerowitz is correct. All nutrients necessary for life are contained in seeds—a food category that includes grain kernels, beans, legumes, and nuts. Because sprouts are so fresh, and do not sit for days or weeks in warehouses, we know that we are getting optimum nutrition.

GREAT WAYS TO SERVE SPROUTS

- Add to tossed salads.
- Use in coleslaw (cabbage, clover, radish).
- Try in wraps and roll-ups (alfalfa, sunflower, radish).
- Stir-fry with other vegetables (alfalfa, clover, radish, mung bean, lentil).
- Blend with vegetable juices (cabbage, mung bean, lentil).
- Mix with soft cheeses, tofu, yogurt, or kefir for a dip (mung bean, radish).
- Stir into soups or stews when serving (mung bean, lentil).
- Eat fresh and uncooked in a sprout salad (salad mixes).
- Top omelets or scrambled eggs (alfalfa, clover, radish).
- Combine in oat, barley, or buckwheat dishes (fenugreek, lentil, mung bean).
- Add to sushi (radish, sunflower).
- Sauté with onions (mung bean, clover, radish).
- Puree with dried peas or beans (mung bean, lentil).
- Add to baked beans (lentil).

WHERE TO FIND SPROUTING SUPPLIES

Inexpensive sprouting kits and seeds are available online and at some health food stores and supermarkets. Buy only certified organic seeds, grains, legumes, or beans for sprouting, purchase them in small quantities, and keep them refrigerated prior to sprouting.

A partial list of seeds, beans, legumes, and grains appropriate for sprouting includes alfalfa, cabbage, clover, fenugreek, mustard, radish, sesame, sunflower, adzuki beans, chickpeas, lentils, mung beans, green peas, wheat, rye, and triticale. If you grow your own sprouts, harvest them within four to eight days for maximum enzymatic activity.

When you do not have the time to grow your own sprouts, purchase them at a local fruit and vegetable market, or in the fresh vegetable department of your supermarket. Health food stores that sell produce often offer sprouts as well. Sprouts are fresh when their roots are moist and white and the sprout itself is crisp.

Caution: Regardless of the source, *do not* use seeds that have been treated with a fungicide. Treated seeds are not edible and can be recognized by the coating of pink or green dust on the seed coat. Seeds sold for planting purposes fall under this category. Use only seeds sold for sprouting or eating, not for planting.

Store sprouts in the vegetable crisper of your refrigerator, and use them as soon as possible. Rinsing daily under cold water can extend their life. Mung bean sprouts can be frozen in an airtight bag for several months, if they are to be used in cooking.

Superfood Number 10: Yogurt and Kefir— Probiotic Partners in Health

The origin of fermented foods and cultured milk products goes so far back that it is rumored to predate recorded history. This is perfectly in keeping with my philosophy that the most ancient foods have survived for a reason—they continue to be instrumental to the survival of our species. Fermented and cultured foods may well represent our first experience with what researchers now call "functional" foods— foods that actively promote optimum health.

The fermented foods scientists consider "probiotic" are primarily yogurt and kefir. What are probiotics, and what do they do?

Early in the twentieth century, research by Nobel Prize–winning biologist Dr. Elie Metchnikoff led him to propose the "intoxication theory" of disease. Metchnikoff believed that aging was accelerated by toxins secreted by unfriendly bacteria that putrefy and ferment food in the intestines. He also believed that the harmless bacteria in fermented milk products might explain the longevity of certain ethnic groups—most notably the peoples of the Caucasus Mountains of southern Russia.

Accordingly, Metchnikoff recommended consuming "cultured" foods, such as yogurt, that contain healthful bacteria. His ideas spread rapidly, and in short order both yogurt and the concept underlying probiotics garnered world attention. And because Metchnikoff identified lactic-acid-secreting bacteria as among the most beneficial, these so-called lactobacilli became an early focus of popular efforts to put Metchnikoff's hypothesis into practice. Today, probiotic microbes are routinely fed to livestock, and it is widely accepted that various *Lactobacillus* and *Bifidobacteria* species hold great promise for enhancing human health.

In humans, probiotic microbes help the body's ongoing fight against infectious diseases by competing with the pathogens for food, nutrients, and survival. This is why human breast milk is rich in nutritional factors that foster the growth of bifidobacteria—a beneficial bacterial family that keeps babies' intestinal ecosystems healthy and disease-resistant.

PROBIOTICS VERSUS DISEASE

Preliminary research supports probiotics' potential to prevent or treat many common conditions. (More research is needed, however, so don't rely on probiotics to help treat any health condition without medical supervision.) Probiotics:

- Ameliorate vaginal (bacterial and yeast), urinary tract, and bladder infections.

- Ameliorate inflammatory intestinal disorders, including inflammatory bowel disease.
- Ameliorate food allergies and inflammatory allergic conditions such as asthma and eczema.
- Reduce several risk factors for cardiovascular disease.
- Reduce several risk factors for intestinal cancers.
- Reduce the duration of gastroenteritis and rotavirus-induced diarrhea in infants.
- Reduce the rate of childhood respiratory infections.
- Ameliorate microbe-induced traveler's diarrhea.
- Help prevent tooth decay.

PROBIOTICS, INFLAMMATION, AND IMMUNE FUNCTION

Researchers have found that people whose diet is rich in probiotic foods enjoy enhanced immune function. It appears that probiotics normalize immune responses, inhibit chronic inflammation, and may improve inflammatory conditions with an autoimmune component, such as asthma, eczema, and Crohn's disease.

Today, there is an alarming emergence of disease-causing agents (viral, bacterial, and more) that are resistant to antibiotics. These dire and potentially life-threatening circumstances have prompted urgent research into the use of probiotic bacteria to battle infections. We now know that probiotics can raise antibody levels in the body. This immune system boost reduces the risk of infections taking hold in the first place, thus avoiding the need for antibiotics. Many doctors recommend live yogurt for patients on antibiotics to replenish good bacteria; some argue that yogurt live cultures may also reduce the occurrence of colds, allergies, and hay fever.

YOGURT VERSUS OBESITY

A daily dose of yogurt is good for people of all ages. Yogurt is also important for those wanting to lose weight. As a milk product, yogurt is naturally rich in calcium. Research shows that calcium helps reduce weight gain. Even small changes in the calcium levels of fat cells can change signals within the cell that control the making and burning of fat.

The authors of a 2003 study at the University of Tennessee placed thirty-four obese people on a low-calorie diet. Sixteen of them were given 400 to 500 mg of calcium in the form of a daily supplement. The other eighteen people ate a diet higher in calcium—1,100 mg per day—in the form of yogurt. After twelve weeks, both groups lost fat. The supplement-taking group had six pounds less fat, but the yogurt group lost about ten pounds of fat. And those who ate yogurt discovered that their waists *shrank by more than an inch and a half.* In comparison, the supplement-taking subjects lost only about a quarter inch in waist size. Finally, a whopping 60 percent of the yogurt eaters' weight loss was belly fat, while only 26 percent of the supplement group's loss was belly fat.

This is very exciting news because belly fat—which we physicians call visceral or intra-abdominal fat—is linked to high cholesterol, high insulin, high triglycerides, high blood pressure, and other problems. Visceral fat may also secrete more disease-linked inflammatory molecules than other types of fat.

The study also reported that in addition to the participants losing more weight, the group that ate yogurt was about twice as effective at maintaining lean muscle mass. As the study director, Michael Zemel, Ph.D., stated in a news release, "This is a critical issue when dieting. You want to lose fat, not muscle. Muscle helps burn calories, but it is often compromised during weight loss." I couldn't agree more!

Always buy organic yogurt, and avoid yogurt that contains thickeners and stabilizers. Also avoid yogurt that contains added sugars or sweetened fruit; these upset the delicate chemical balance that allows the cultures to thrive. Sugars also feed the growth of unwanted yeasts, such as *Candida albicans.*

KEFIR: ANCIENT ELIXIR

I start every morning by pouring myself a glass of unsweetened whole-milk kefir and add to it two tablespoons of POM Wonderful (pure pomegranate extract). I stir it up, and it looks and tastes like a rich and beautiful berry smoothie. It is the perfect way to start the day.

Kefir (*kee*-fer) is a fermented, probiotic milk drink from the Caucasus Mountains in the former Soviet Union. The name *kefir* loosely translated means "pleasure" or "good feeling." Due to its health-promoting properties, kefir was once considered a gift from the gods. Fortunately, it is being rediscovered and recognized for its many health and beauty benefits.

Kefir can best be described as a sort of liquid, sparkling yogurt, with its own distinct and deliciously mild, naturally sweet, yet tangy flavor—with a refreshing hint of natural carbonation. Its unique taste and almost mystical reputation as a longevity elixir explain why people all over Europe are making kefir (along with similar fermented drinks) their beverage of choice. Sales are even beginning to rival top soft drink brands. Unlike yogurt, which is created from milk by adding certain lactic acid bacteria, kefir is made by combining milk with a pinch of "kefir grains"—the folk term coined to describe a complex mixture of yeasts and lactobacillus bacteria. The small amount of carbon dioxide, alcohol, and aromatic compounds produced by the cultures gives kefir its distinct fizzy, tangy taste.

Kefir also contains unique polysaccharides (long-chain sugars) called kefiran, which may be responsible for some of its health benefits. Much of the Russian research on its health benefits remains untranslated, and Western research is in its early stages—but the results to date support kefir's impressive folk reputation.

This mildly self-carbonated beverage is popular in the Caucasus, Russia, and southwestern Asia, and recently gained wide popularity in Western Europe. In the United States, most natural food stores and the "whole food" chain markets found in urban areas—such as Whole Foods Market and Wild Oats—carry kefir. Given the ever-increasing popularity of yogurt and yogurt drinks here, I predict it won't be long before the big U.S. supermarket chains follow suit. However, as with yogurt, beware of products laden with sugars and fructose. Buy plain, unsweetened kefir and flavor with mixed berries, including açaí.

KEFIR'S HEALTH BENEFITS

In addition to kefir's ancient reputation as a healthy drink, it has been famously credited with the extraordinary longevity of people in the Caucasus. Hospitals in the former Soviet Union use kefir—especially when no modern medical treatment is available—to treat conditions ranging from atherosclerosis, allergic disease, metabolic and digestive disorders, and tuberculosis to cancer and gastrointestinal disorders.

A number of studies conducted to date have documented kefir's ability to stimulate the immune system, enhance lactose digestion, and inhibit tumors, fungi, and pathogens—including the bacteria that cause most ulcers. This makes a lot of sense, because scientists have since discovered that most ulcers are caused by an infection with the bacterium *Helicobacter pylori* and *not* by spicy food, stomach acid, or stress, as physicians erroneously believed for years.

Scientists are now discovering that a great many inflammatory diseases (including certain types of heart disease) can be triggered by a bacterium. And that provides all the more reason to enjoy kefir as part of your daily diet.

The next chapter explores the exotic world of spices, unlocking their secrets to longevity and ageless beauty. Just tiny amounts of these remarkable foods can dramatically change the way you look and feel, in addition to greatly increasing the flavor, digestibility, and palatability of your favorite foods.

5 Spices of Life

Are you going to Scarborough Fair?
Parsley, sage, rosemary, and thyme . . .
Remember me to one who lived there . . .
She once was a true love of mine.

— ANONYMOUS, THIRTEENTH- TO
FIFTEENTH-CENTURY ENGLAND

SOMETIMES THE SOLUTION TO A PROBLEM hides in plain sight. Modern science seeks ways to reduce the deterioration of the mind and body that accompanies aging. So far, efforts to slow aging or help prevent the specific diseases of aging have borne little fruit. One reason for this is the failure of our health care system to address basic facts such as the role of our diet in health, longevity, and disease. Instead we now face an epidemic of obesity, with all of its resultant diseases (diabetes, Syndrome X, heart disease . . .), beginning in childhood. Until we recognize that our "fast-food nation" is on the fast track to early death and disease, all the magic bullets in the world aren't going to help us. For example, while statin drugs reduce cholesterol levels, none has been shown to substantially reduce the risk of heart attack. And the consensus of experts is that the drugs now available to treat Alzheimer's disease offer such slim benefits as to constitute an annual waste of $1.2 billion.

One reason for these failures is that science focuses almost exclusively on the minutiae of basic biomedical research. While this work is useful in the long term, the near-total focus on basic research distracts us from exploring the strong anti-aging and preventive-health promise of common foods. I believe we already possess persuasive evidence that successful anti-aging efforts start with the rainbow foods and superfoods described in chapters 3 and 4. When we recognize that inflammation is the basis of accelerated aging and accompanying degenerative diseases, this makes perfect sense. Treat the body holistically, starting with the foods we eat, to prevent inflammation on a cellular level. No drug or therapy can be more effective. We need to work with the body, to strengthen and revitalize all organ systems, which means that our "cures" need to be *physiologic*—that is, in accord with or characteristic of the normal functioning of a living organism.

While the rainbow and superfoods are central to any anti-aging anti-inflammatory strategy, certain other plant foods pack even more anti-aging punch, pound for pound. I'm talking about an overlooked part of most people's diets: the herbs and spices in your pantry. The very familiarity of common culinary herbs and spices serves to obscure their potential as anti-aging powerhouses. While scientists only began probing their biochemical properties about twenty years ago, it's already clear that ounce for ounce, many herbs and spices offer tremendous anti-aging potential, thanks to these flavorings' unsurpassed antioxidant, anti-inflammatory capacities.

What I find so exciting about these different classes of foods is that, in addition to their extremely powerful antioxidant effects, a number of these foods, herbs, and spices possess unique properties that can enhance *insulin sensitivity* while decreasing *cortisol levels*. This is extremely important because as the body ages, we see changes that include the loss of muscle tone in conjunction with the addition of body fat, particularly in the abdominal area, on the legs, and on the arms. This excess body fat is directly attributable to two factors. The first is the loss of insulin sensitivity, the second the elevation of cortisol (the death hormone) levels in conjunction with a decrease in the life or youth hormones, testosterone, estrogen, human growth hormone, and so on.

Culinary Herbs: Tasty, Aromatic Anti-Aging Aids

In 1966, the folk-rock duo Simon & Garfunkel scored a hit single with an old English folk song, "Scarborough Fair," whose famous refrain—"parsley, sage, rosemary, and thyme"—also served as the title of their best-selling album. It's likely that few of the group's fans knew that these common culinary herbs were once prized throughout Europe as important drugs and health tonics. In fact, until the advent of modern drugs, parsley, sage, rosemary, and thyme—and companion herbs such as lavender, mint, and oregano—were key tools of the herbal doctors who preceded today's more scientific physicians. It is no wonder that the world was singing (and continues to sing) their praises!

During the sixteenth-century reign of Queen Elizabeth I—when doctors were scarce, expensive, and of dubious utility for treating most illnesses—the encyclopedic plant medicine guides known as herbals occupied a place second only to the Bible in literate households. These works, such as the famous herbal encyclopedia by Nicholas Culpepper, distilled knowledge transmitted down the centuries from India, China, Persia, Greece, and Rome.

IS IT AN HERB OR A SPICE?

In this chapter, you'll see both terms used. In general, *herbs* are fragrant plants used in flavoring various foods and/or for medicinal purposes. *Spices* are dried, aromatic plants used for flavoring foods, for medicinal purposes, and sometimes as food preservatives. In many cultures, the words *herb* and *spice* are interchangeable.

Remember what I said in the last chapter: Although many herbs and spices have reported medical benefits, if you have any type of health problem or physical symptom, *do not self-diagnose or self-medicate.* Trust your medical professional first and foremost in this department.

In recent decades, the U.S. Department of Agriculture (USDA) has pioneered research into the antioxidant powers of common fruits and vegetables. Working with researchers at Tufts University, USDA scientists have begun to compile unprecedented information on the power of plant foods to neutralize the negative effects of free radicals. Using the oxygen radical absorbance capacity (ORAC) scale, described in chapter 3, the USDA/Tufts team has begun to document what traditional healers discovered after centuries of trial and error: that common culinary herbs pack immense preventive-health power.

In fact, it turns out that many of the everyday, seemingly unremarkable herbs in people's pantries pack unsurpassed antioxidant power. In 2001, for example, USDA scientists published their research into twenty-seven culinary herbs and twelve medicinal herbs. The study revealed that many common culinary herbs exert free-radical-quenching capacities higher than those reported for the berries and vegetables long considered the antioxidant champs. In other words, small amounts of these herbs supply the same amount of antioxidants found in much larger amounts of fruits or vegetables.

Let's take a closer look at the antioxidant champions in our pantries, on our windowsills, and in our herb gardens.

ANTIOXIDANT CAPACITY* OF 25 COMMON HERBS

Remember that the ORAC scores for culinary herbs appear to be much lower than the ORAC scores for fruits and vegetables (see Rainbow Foods, chapter 3) when, in fact, culinary herbs have more antioxidant content and capacity per ounce. This is because different researchers use different, noncomparable measuring scales.

RANK	ORAC SCORE
1. Southwest oregano** *(Poliomintha longiflora)*	92.18
2. Italian oregano*** *(Origanum x majoricum)*	71.64
3. Greek oregano *(Origanum vulgare* subsp. *hirtum)*	64.71

Rank	ORAC Score
4. Sweet (European) bay leaf	31.70
5. Dill	29.12
6. Winter savory *(Satureja montana)*	26.34
7. Vietnamese coriander	22.90
8. Orange mint	19.80
9. Garden thyme *(Thymus vulgaris)*	19.49
10. *Ginkgo biloba*	19.18
11. Rosemary	19.15
12. Lemon verbena	17.88
13. Saint-John's-wort	16.77
14. English lavender	16.20
15. Valerian	15.82
16. Sweet basil	14.27
17. Creeping thyme	13.40
18. Lemon thyme	13.28
19. Garden sage *(Salvia officinalis)*	12.28
20. Pineapple sage	11.55
21. Parsley	11.03
22. Caraway	10.65
23. Chive	9.15
24. Spearmint	8.10
25. Fennel	5.88

*Zheng W, Wang SY. Antioxidant activity and phenolic compounds in selected herbs. J Agric Food Chem. 2001 Nov;49(11):5165-70. ORAC values are expressed as micromoles of Trolox (synthetic vitamin E analogue) equivalents per gram of fresh weight.

**Southwest oregano *(P. longiflora* or *P. bustamanta)* leaf is not usually sold in the United States, but seed suppliers may be able to find it for you to plant. It is often confused with Mexican oregano *(Lippia graveolens)*, a completely different plant that is available in the U.S. Reportedly, Mexican oregano is high in carvacrol and should therefore be high in antioxidant power. Spanish thyme (Cuban oregano) is not a true member of the oregano family, offers a strong, oregano-like flavor, and is likely to possess substantial antioxidant power.

***Also known as hardy sweet marjoram, this pungent, peppery herb is a cross between Greek oregano *(O. vulgare* subsp. *hirtum)* and sweet marjoram *(O. majorana)*.

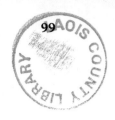

Exploring the Antioxidant Herbs

OREGANO

The culinary herbs with the highest ORAC scores are three types of oregano. Each one's antioxidant capacities are much higher than that of vitamin E, a potent antioxidant that is used for comparison values on the ORAC scale.

Oregano is both the scientific name for the genus that encompasses various members of the larger mint (Lamiaceae) family, and a folk term that refers to any of a wide range of unrelated plants with "oregano-like" fragrances and flavors. A great deal of confusion surrounds the very similar herbs known as oregano and marjoram, but all marjoram plants are members of the genus *Origanum,* and they share an overlapping set of antioxidant compounds and fragrant essential oils (a misnomer, by the way, since these are not fats or oils).

In Greek, *oregano* means "mountain joy," and it is, fittingly, Greek oregano that is the best-tasting and most widely used variety. All of the various types of oregano share the unique flavor and scent characteristic of the antioxidant phenol called carvacrol (cymophenol), which is also found in thyme, savory, caraway, and sweet marjoram. Just as capsaicin is the common, healthful thread that binds all types of peppers—sweet and chili—it is carvacrol that makes oregano such a savory, pungent, warming herb. Oregano also contains high levels of rosmarinic acid, which occurs in rosemary and several other strongly antioxidant herbs.

Health Benefits of Oregano

- The thymol and carvacrol in oregano inhibit the growth of bacteria, and are more effective against the *Giardia* parasite (a cause of many cases of "traveler's diarrhea") than the commonly used prescription drug.
- Ounce for ounce, oregano's antioxidant capacity is forty-two times greater than that of apples, twelve times greater than that of oranges, and four times greater than that of blueberries.

- Oregano is a good source of iron, vitamin A, dietary fiber, calcium, manganese, magnesium, and vitamin B_6.

Cooking Tips

Prized for its peppery leaves, oregano adds a unique flavor note to Italian tomato sauces and diverse Mediterranean dishes. As a woody perennial, oregano usually survives through the Northern winter, and makes an indispensable addition to any backyard or window-box herb garden. Italian oregano, also known as hardy sweet marjoram—a cross between Greek oregano and sweet marjoram—is both sweet and savory, and is good with meats, eggs, soups, and vegetables.

BAY LEAF

European (sweet) bay leaf is a member of the same family as cinnamon, cassia, sassafras, and avocado, and boasts a complex blend of fragrances and flavors, from balsam to citrus. The bay, or laurel, leaf was famous in ancient Greece and Rome, where heroes from emperors to poets wore wreaths of laurel leaves. We still associate this plant with achievement and honor when we name someone poet laureate. And *baccalaureate,* which signifies the completion of a bachelor's degree, means "laurel berries."

Health Benefits of Bay Leaves

Bay leaves and berries:

- Improve digestion.
- Are an astringent, which means they help contract tissues or canals in the body and therefore diminish discharges such as mucus and blood.
- Help relieve gas.

Cooking Tips

Bay leaves are used throughout the world in soups, sauces, and stews and are an appropriate seasoning for fish, meat, and poultry. Bay leaves are often included among pickling spices. Mediterranean cooks traditionally add the leaves to sauces, removing them before serving.

DILL: HEALTH BENEFITS

The main phytonutrients in dill activate the potent antioxidant enzyme glutathione-S-transferase, which helps attach the molecule glutathione to oxidized molecules that would otherwise damage the body. This activity helps protect against carcinogens such as those found in cigarette smoke, charcoal grill smoke, trash incinerator smoke, therapeutic drugs, and products of oxidative stress. Pretty important stuff for something usually relegated to the pickle barrel!

Cooking Tips

Famous as a flavoring for pickles, this feathery member of the carrot family also complements fish, chicken and chicken soup, and even yogurt. Fresh dill freezes well.

LEMON BALM

Lemon balm has a long history. The Roman scholar Pliny and the Greek physician Dioscorides both used lemon balm as a medicinal herb. In the sixteenth century, herbalist John Gerard gave lemon balm to students to "quicken the senses." The American colonists used lemon balm, and it was noted that Thomas Jefferson grew it in his garden at Monticello.

Health Benefits of Lemon Balm

New research indicates that, like rosemary, lemon balm helps people learn, store, and retrieve information. Laboratory tests have found that lemon balm, like the nutrient dimethylaminoethanol (DMAE), increased the activity of acetylcholine—a chemical messenger essential to memory and other cognitive functions, which is reduced in people with Alzheimer's disease.

Cooking Tips

Lemon balm makes a light, lemony tea, and is a delightful addition to fish, mushrooms, and soft cheeses. Fresh leaves are used in salads, marinades (especially for vegetables), chicken salad, and poultry stuffing.

SPICY TIDBITS

Here are some interesting facts about a few of the spices in this chapter.

Cardamom. If you've ever been in a Starbucks (and who hasn't?), you know that one of its most popular noncoffee offerings is chai tea, a spiced tea from India. The most common flavorings in chai are cardamom, cinnamon, cloves, and even black pepper. The most surprising fact about chai is that it is not as common in India as it is in the Western world's ubiquitous coffee shops and Indian restaurants. In fact, spiced tea (chai masala) is, in India, a luxury few can afford every day.

Cinnamon. Cinnamon has been a prized commodity since ancient times; in some eras, it was more precious than gold. When the Roman emperor Nero's wife died, he burned a year's supply of cinnamon on her funeral pyre—a gesture unheard of at the time and meant to signify just how important she had been to him. In 1536, the Portuguese invaded Sri Lanka. The conquerors did not ask for money in tribute—they asked for cinnamon, and for many years a local king paid the Portuguese a tribute of almost a quarter million pounds of cinnamon annually.

Clove. **A small Indonesian island called Ternate, nicknamed Clove Island, has been trading this spice with China for more than two thousand years. In China, cloves were used for cooking, but also as a form of deodorant—all those called in to see the emperor had to chew cloves before they were allowed into his presence.**

MINT: HEALTH BENEFITS

Mint, an ancient symbol of hospitality and purification, is said to be good for colds, flu, and fevers, as well as throat and sinus ailments. Mint tea soothes the stomach, and its aroma has a calming effect.

Cooking Tips

Try tossing cooked eggplant with chopped mint leaves, plain yogurt, garlic, and cayenne, or make a delicious salad by combining fennel, onions, and mint leaves. Chopped mint leaves complement gazpacho and other tomato-based soups. Yogurt dressings, dips, and soups often include mint. Fresh mint is vastly preferable to dried mint, for both its flavor and its health benefits.

THYME

Thymus is a Greek name for "courage"—but in Greek, it also means "to fumigate." Egyptians used thyme as part of the mummification process.

Health Benefits of Thyme

Many of thyme's health benefits are attributed to thymol. Studies have shown that the brain and the major organs benefit because thymol facilitates significantly higher antioxidant enzyme activities and total antioxidant status. This is partly attributed to its ability to protect the omega-3 fatty acids in cell membranes by increasing their proportions relative to other fatty acids.

Thyme contains flavonoids and carvacrol, along with vitamin B complex, vitamin C, and vitamin D. It has been used for medicinal purposes for centuries, for such problems as gastrointestinal ailments, laryngitis, diarrhea, and lack of appetite. It helps reduce fever. It is good for chronic respiratory problems, including colds, flu, bronchitis, and sore throats. It is also good for external use in fighting inflammation and infection, and can be helpful for athlete's foot and shingles.

Cooking Tips

Thyme can be used to flavor soups, fish, meat, poultry, and eggs. It is also ideal in tomato and mushroom sauces. The preferred varieties of thyme are narrow-leafed, strong-flavored French thyme, and milder, broad-leafed English thyme. In Britain, thyme is the most popular culinary herb after mint. In the United States, it is an important ingredient in the Creole cooking of New Orleans, where it is used as part of the spice mix in the blackening cooking technique—which I don't recommend, because foods cooked in this manner promote glycation. In Central America, it is a valued ingredient in making jerk seasoning for poultry and other meats.

PARSLEY: HEALTH BENEFITS

Studies have shown that the flavonoids in parsley—a bright green herb used as both a seasoning and a garnish—function as powerful protection against free radicals. In addition, parsley is an excellent source of vitamin C, beta-carotene, and folic acid.

Cooking Tips

Italian flat-leafed parsley has a stronger flavor than the curly kind, and holds up better in cooking. Parsley should be added near the end of cooking to preserve its taste and nutritional value. Add chopped parsley to pesto (a basil, olive oil, and pine nut sauce) to lighten its flavor, and lend it more texture and phytonutrient power. Combine chopped parsley, garlic, and lemon zest to make a delicious rub for chicken, lamb, and beef. Parsley is great in soups and tomato sauces, and a bit of chopped parsley complements just about every dish, including salads, vegetable sautés, and grilled seafoods.

ROSEMARY

In the Middle Ages, rosemary's apparent ability to fortify the memory transformed it into a symbol of fidelity—it was known as the herb of remembrance—and it was used symbolically in the costumes, decorations, and gifts used at weddings. During the Renaissance, rosemary oil was used to make a very popular cosmetic called Queen of Hungary water.

Health Benefits of Rosemary

Over the years, rosemary became popular as a digestive aid, as an antispasmodic for dysmenorrhea (painful menstruation), and to relieve respiratory disorders. Today, we know that rosemary's phytonutrients do in fact stimulate the immune system, boost circulation, relax smooth muscles of the trachea and intestine, protect and stimulate the liver, inhibit tumor activity, enhance digestion, and help reduce the severity of asthma attacks. And confirming the hard-won wisdom of our ancestors, research has shown that rosemary increases circulation to the head and brain, thereby improving concentration and memory.

The effects of key rosemary phytonutrients—especially caffeic acid derivatives such as rosmarinic acid—are also likely to help ameliorate spasmodic disorders, peptic ulcer, inflammatory diseases, atherosclerosis, ischemic heart disease, cataracts, and certain cancers. In addition to rosemary, rosmarinic acid is found in large amounts in lemon balm, the mints, marjoram, and sage.

Cooking Tips

Rosemary's heady, piney aroma makes it the perfect seasoning for roasted meats, especially lamb. You can also add fresh rosemary to omelets and frittatas, and use it to season chicken and tomato sauces or soups.

MORE SPICY TIDBITS

Cumin. We know that cumin was used in ancient times because cumin seeds have been found in Egyptian pyramids. The Greeks and Romans used it for medicinal purposes, but they also used it cosmetically to induce a pallid complexion. Also during that time, cumin came to symbolize greed. In fact, the emperor Marcus Aurelius (who was famous for his avarice) was called Cuminus behind his back.

Dill. The word *dill* comes from the Norse *dilla,* meaning "to lull." For hundreds of years, dill tea was used to help insomniacs get a good night's sleep. In medieval Europe, it was used in love potions and to ward off spells (you could protect yourself from witchcraft by wearing a bag of dried dill over your heart). A seventeenth-century epic poem called "Nymphidia" by Michael Drayton includes the lines "Therewith her Veruayne and her Dill, That hindreth Witches of their will."

Fenugreek. The Latin name for this herb means "Greek hay"; the dried plant smells very much like a bale of hay.

SAGE: HEALTH BENEFITS

Like its close cousin rosemary, sage contains a variety of essential oils, flavonoids, antioxidant enzymes, and phenolic acids, including the rosmarinic acid found in rosemary and other culinary herbs. Rosmarinic acid curbs inflammation by reducing production of inflammatory peptides such as leukotriene B4, and through its strong antioxidant effects. Sage may therefore alleviate inflammatory conditions such as rheumatoid arthritis, bronchial asthma, diabetes, and atherosclerosis.

And like rosemary, sage enhances memory and concentration. In fact, the dried root of Chinese sage *(Salvia miltiorrhiza)* has been used for hundreds of years to treat brain dysfunction, and modern research shows that it contains phytonutrients resembling the synthetic acetyl-choline esterase inhibitor drugs used to treat Alzheimer's disease.

Cooking Tips

Like rosemary, sage emits a pleasant, pine-like aroma. It's a common ingredient in poultry stuffing, and is traditionally used in sausage, helping to keep it fresh. Sage is also a traditional "purifying" herb—Native Americans burn bunches of sage to purify sacred spaces—and folk mouthwash ingredient.

BASIL

Basil, one of the most popular herbs in America, was virtually unknown outside Europe thirty years ago. Today, due to improved dehydration and shipping techniques, it is enjoyed everywhere.

Health Benefits of Basil

The flavonoids in basil protect cell structures and chromosomes from radiation and free radicals. Basil reduces unwanted bacterial growth, thanks to its aromatic essential oils. Basil inhibits the growth of food-borne disease bacteria—some of which are resistant to common antibiotics—including *Listeria, Staphylococcus,* and *E. coli.* Washing produce in a 1 percent solution of basil or thyme essential oil virtually eliminates dangerous shigella bacteria. Adding fresh thyme or basil to vinaigrette will make salads tastier while helping ensure that they are safer to eat. Basil's essential oil, eugenol, blocks the inflammatory cyclooxygenase (COX) enzymes, the same ones blocked by synthetic nonsteroidal anti-inflammatory drugs such as aspirin and ibuprofen. This means that basil has anti-aging powers and may even help alleviate the symptoms of inflammatory health problems such as rheumatoid arthritis, diabetes, or inflammatory bowel conditions.

Basil is also good for your heart. It is also high in beta-carotene, which protects the lining of blood vessels from free-radical damage and helps prevent them from oxidizing cholesterol in the blood, thus inhibiting the development of atherosclerosis and reducing the risk of heart attacks and strokes. As a good source of vitamin B_6, basil may help reduce blood levels of homocysteine, excess amounts of which damage blood vessel walls. And basil is a good source of magnesium, which relaxes blood vessels, improves blood flow, and reduces the risk of irregular heart rhythms or spasms.

Cooking Tips

Basil is delicious on chicken, fish, pasta, stews, salads, and vegetables. Add basil in the last ten minutes of cooking; heat will dissipate its strong, rich flavor. When possible, add fresh basil to salads—it is especially complementary when served with fresh tomatoes.

EVEN SPICIER TIDBITS

Garlic has long been prized for its medicinal properties. Egyptian pyramid builders were given garlic every day to keep them healthy. In France, garlic is sometimes known as *thériaque des pauvres*, which means "theriac of the poor," after a medieval medicinal mixture called theriac, which only the rich could afford. The poor had to make do with garlic. And of course, garlic is the weapon of choice in the fight against vampires. Romanians used to smear garlic on all windows and entrances to their houses and land, and made certain that they ate garlic every day for their protection. They also placed garlic in a corpse's mouth to prevent evil spirits from entering the dead body.

Oregano. Although oregano has been used for centuries in Europe, it was virtually unknown in America until after World War II. It came into its own when pizza was introduced to this country. Pizza began as a meal for the poor; it was little more than a piece of bread with tomato paste on top. In 1889, when King Umberto and Queen Margherita of Italy traveled to Naples, a local baker added white mozzarella cheese and green basil leaves to the red tomato paste (giving the dish the colors of the Italian flag). This became known as Pizza Margherita and soon became popular around the world. Today, pizza doesn't usually include basil, but it does include oregano. For obvious reasons, pizza is not a dish I recommend as part of your daily diet, but an occasional slice can be delicious.

Add Spice to Your Life: Anti-Aging Allies from the Indies

In school, we all learned about the Age of Exploration, and that the demand for spices was the prime purpose of its heroes' epic voyages. Europeans of the Middle Ages eagerly sought supplies of pepper, nutmeg, cinnamon, cloves, and other spices, both to enhance their bland fare and to preserve meats in the dark days before ice markets and then electricity enabled refrigeration.

Arab traders first brought Asia's exotic spices overland to the European market, which paid enormous premiums for these exotic culinary treasures. While Columbus and company never neglected to seek gold in unknown lands, they mainly strove to establish direct trade links to the Asian sources of costly spices.

As soon as advances in navigation and sailing technology allowed, European mariners set out for India, Java, and Sumatra, determined to cut out the middlemen and keep spice profits for themselves. At the time, Asian spices were almost literally worth their weight in gold to the courageous captains who managed to get them back home.

Today, most spices are quite inexpensive. They remain as valuable as they were in the Age of Exploration, however, but for even better reasons: their anti-aging and preventive-health powers. Many of the spices we associate with curry—or with seasonal fare such as mulled cider or pumpkin pie—do much more than just add flavor and zest to foods.

Our ancestors knew that spices could help preserve foods. What they couldn't know is the how and the why. Cloves, cinnamon, turmeric, cardamom, fenugreek, mustard, nutmeg, licorice, and ginger preserve foods because they are rich in antioxidants.

Although there are thousands of spices in the world, the rest of this chapter will focus on two closely related spices in particular—ginger and turmeric—that exert especially powerful antioxidant and anti-inflammatory effects and that, in their most potent, fresh form, lend themselves to frequent use in cooking.

Both of these remarkable anti-aging, healing plants belong to the same botanical family (Zingiberaceae) as "Thai ginger," or galangal, with which they share many active compounds. The parts of the turmeric and ginger plants used for cooking and medicine, which are called roots, are actually rhizomes—the tuberous root of flowering plants. The following facts should explain why I urge my patients to include plenty of turmeric and ginger in their household menus.

Ginger: A Root of Health

To many of us, our sole relationship whith ginger was in our childhood fondness for ginger ale, gingerbread, or gingersnaps. Little did we realize that ginger is actually a powerful anti-aging remedy—an amazingly effective anti-inflammatory food with many health benefits and no side effects, and a very long medicinal tradition throughout the Eastern world. As is often the case, research into ginger's multifaceted anti-aging and health attributes is limited, and not well known to the public or scientists in the West—although this is rapidly changing. And sad to say, the familiarity of common foods with health-promoting properties fails to attract pharmaceutical company research, which seeks out single plant compounds, synthetic versions of which can be marketed as highly profitable, patent-protected drugs. Unfortunately, this approach ignores the synergistic and additive effects of the many phytonutrients in herbs and spices, which generally work better—and more safely—together than alone.

Ginger has a long list of medicinal purposes. For instance, it has a traditional reputation—now clinically proven—as an anti-nausea remedy effective in treating both motion and morning sickness. Nonetheless, people think they have to buy pharmaceutical anti-nausea drugs with adverse side effects, even though these drugs are generally no more effective than ginger. Ginger greatly aids digestion of protein, thanks to an enzyme called zingibain that matches the protein-digesting power of the papaya enzyme papain found in most meat tenderizers. According to researcher Paul Schulick, author of *Ginger: Common Spice & Wonder Drug,* gingerroot is so rich in zingibain that one pound matches the protein-digesting power of 180 pounds of papaya—and unlike papaya, ginger does not rate high on the glycemic index. Zingibain also dissolves the immune complexes that precipitate the symptoms of rheumatoid arthritis.

As an anti-inflammatory, ginger is as effective as nonsteroidal anti-inflammatory drugs (NSAIDs) such as aspirin—with none of their dangerous side effects. In fact, ginger shines as a preventive-health powerhouse that safely derails inflammatory processes in several ways.

HOW DO I TAKE GINGER?

Aside from using fresh ginger in cooking, to make tea, or adding it to fruit or vegetable blender drinks, you can also take supplemental ginger. Let's look at the pros and cons of each form:

- Fresh ginger contains more of the rhizome's anti-inflammatory gingerol compounds than dried. In fragrance tests, fresh ginger can be detected in dilutions as low as one part in thirty-five thousand, while dried ginger cannot be detected until it reaches one part in fifteen hundred to two thousand.
- Ginger extracts—available in either a dropper bottle or in capsules—concentrate the active constituents of fresh ginger in smaller amounts. While my first choice is fresh ginger, extracts offer a convenient, practical alternative means for getting large

amounts of ginger's active compounds without having to eat large quantities of ginger. Extracts may contain small amounts of the alcohol used to extract the rhizome's active principles. A new method called supercritical extraction employs carbon dioxide instead of alcohol, and produces extracts roughly comparable in quality.

- Dried ginger contains higher concentrations of the analgesic shogaol compounds found in fresh ginger. It comes in capsules at the healthstore or drugstore—or you can save money by buying it in bulk from health food or gourmet stores. Look for organic ginger to minimize intake of pesticide residues.

GINGER: A SAFETY NOTE

Ginger is an ancient, time-honored food and tonic, commonly prescribed worldwide for cold symptom relief, motion sickness, and upset stomach. Among common medicinal foods and herbs, it is now one of the top three most heavily researched, and ginger is considered safe by all U.S. regulatory agencies.

Arthritis researchers in Denmark reported no side effects among participants in any of their many test subjects, who consumed 3 to 50 grams (0.1 to 1.8 ounces) of ginger per day for more than two years. That said, taking more than 1 or 2 grams on an empty stomach is likely to produce a brief, harmless burning sensation.

However, ginger increases menstrual flow when taken in extremely large quantities. Physicians advise against taking more than 1 to 2 grams per day during the first trimester of pregnancy. Use moderation in all things, and consult with your physician before taking significant amounts of ginger if you are on blood-thinning drugs, have any disease symptoms, or are pregnant.

GINGER AND TURMERIC FOR
HEART HEALTH

Both ginger and turmeric help reduce the risk of cardio-vascular disease in at least four ways:

1. **Slow the development of sclerotic lesions, which lead to clogged, inflamed arteries.**
2. **Significantly reduce blood levels of LDL (bad) cholesterol and its susceptibility to damaging oxidation and clumping.**
3. **Counter the tendency of blood platelets to clump in the presence of pro-inflammatory stimuli.**
4. **Reduce blood pressure.**

TURMERIC: THE GOLD STANDARD

Turmeric is an Indian curry spice with an ancient history of medicinal use against inflammation. This delicious spice—most familiar as the brilliant golden-yellow color in curry powder—is a close cousin to ginger, and has been used for millennia to flavor, color, and preserve foods.

To the ancient Aryan peoples of South Asia, who worshiped the sun, turmeric was prized for its sun-like golden-yellow dye. Since time immemorial, married Indian women have applied turmeric to their cheeks in the evening, in anticipation of a visit by Lakshmi—the goddess of good fortune. This custom, still practiced in some parts of India, is probably a remnant of the ancient sun-worshiping tradition.

The almost iridescent yellow color of turmeric has enjoyed broad use as a dye for cotton, silk, paper, wood, foods, and cosmetics, and as a food preservative. Long used by India's ayurvedic physicians to treat gastrointestinal and inflammatory ailments, turmeric is also applied cosmetically to enhance skin health and tone. Topical turmeric-based ointments are used in India to treat joint pain, bruises, and a wide variety of skin disorders, including infections, inflammation, blemishes, wounds, acne, boils, burns, and eczema.

The significance of turmeric to modern medicine became apparent after the discovery of its potent antioxidant properties, most of which derive from curcumin, the common name for turmeric's yellow polyphenol pigments, which scientists refer to as curcuminoids. Even though they constitute only about 5 percent of turmeric powder, curcuminoids give turmeric much of its amazing anti-inflammatory, antioxidant power.

Antioxidant Attributes of Turmeric

- The curcuminoid pigments in turmeric are safe, highly effective antioxidants. In fact, turmeric's curcuminoids may prevent oxidation of blood fats better than the OPCs in pine bark and grape seed extracts, or the strong synthetic antioxidant BHT, based on test-tube studies.
- Turmeric contains a unique peptide called turmerin, a free-radical scavenger that is more powerful than curcumin or the potent synthetic antioxidant BHA.
- Animals fed curcuminoids show higher blood levels of the enzyme glutathione-S-transferase, an important antioxidant and key player in the body's detoxification system.

Anti-Inflammatory Powers of Turmeric

Like ginger, curcumin may be a much safer anti-inflammatory agent than standard NSAIDs such as aspirin and ibuprofen. Turmeric sensitizes the body's cortisol receptor sites, and its anti-inflammatory properties are considered comparable to those of the body's own cortisone-type hormones. This is of critical importance to the Perricone Promise: We must keep our cortisol levels low to prevent accelerated aging of all organ systems—including the skin.

ANTI-CANCER ATTRIBUTES OF TURMERIC

Researchers at the University of California, San Diego, reported that "Curcumin should be considered as a safe, non-toxic and easy-to-use chemotherapeutic agent for colorectal cancers." Human clinical trials show it is nontoxic at doses of up to 10 grams (one-third ounce) per day. All of the many dozens of studies conducted to date in the United States and beyond suggest that turmeric—and especially its curcumin fraction—possesses enormous potential in the prevention and treatment of cancer.

Turmeric also enhances the liver's ability to eliminate dangerous carcinogenic toxins. A recent study demonstrated that dietary turmeric can raise the levels of two very important liver detoxification enzymes, UDP glucuronyl transferase and glutathione-S-transferase. As the researchers reported, "The results suggest that turmeric may increase detoxification systems in addition to its antioxidant properties. . . . Turmeric used widely as a spice would probably mitigate the effects of several dietary carcinogens."

One other note on this topic: Making classic lentil or bean dishes seasoned and flavored with turmeric will give you extra protection from colon cancer thanks to the high fiber in the lentils and beans and the antioxidant abilities of the turmeric.

TURMERIC FOR CARDIOVASCULAR HEALTH

Curcumin helps prevent oxidation of cholesterol in the blood, which damages blood vessels and builds up in the plaque that can lead to heart attack or stroke. Turmeric is also high in vitamin B_6, which keeps levels of homocysteine from getting too high, a major risk factor for cardiovascular disease; ample intake of vitamin B_6 seems to reduce that risk.

TURMERIC FOR BRAIN AND NERVES

Population studies in India show that elderly people whose diets are high in turmeric enjoy low levels of neurological diseases such as

Alzheimer's. Alzheimer's disease is considered an inflammatory condition, and physicians who researched curcumin's preventive and therapeutic properties at the University of California, Los Angeles, came away impressed. As they reported, "In view of its efficacy and apparent low toxicity, this Indian spice component shows promise for the prevention of Alzheimer's disease." In particular, curcumin is a strong inducer of the "heat-shock-protein response," which protects cells from oxidative damage, and may be a key component of Alzheimer's disease.

Preliminary studies also suggest that curcumin may block the progression of multiple sclerosis (MS), possibly by reducing the production of the IL-2 protein that destroys the myelin sheath protecting most nerves in the body. Loss of myelin is a key factor in MS.

HOW CAN I GET MORE TURMERIC IN MY DIET?

The simple answer is "enjoy curry often," because the many variations of this zesty, versatile seasoning mix go well with many meats, vegetables, and certain fish, and also contain several other healthful spices. That said, there are a few considerations when it comes to getting turmeric into your body:

- While commercial curry powders are probably fairly low in active constituents, frequent use probably confers significant benefit. Commercial curry pastes are likely higher in active constituents, but some are very high in fat and calories (check the label). You can also mix up your own curry powder, varying the ingredients to suit your taste. Store in the freezer to protect volatile oils. Pure turmeric powder is often available at natural food stores.
- Unlike ginger, fresh turmeric is usually found only in Southeast Asian and Indian markets. Like fresh ginger, fresh turmeric probably has more active constituents than the dried root. (Be careful when handling fresh turmeric—it can stain your hands and clothes.) And as with ginger, in addition to liberal use in soups, stews, and lentil and bean dishes, I recommend taking

extracts—alcohol or supercritical carbon dioxide type—for maximum potency and convenience.

Turmeric's Spicy Sidekicks

When it comes to curry, turmeric may be the antioxidant king, but it's not the only valuable spice in this classic seasoning, or in your cabinet. Most curries contain cardamom, turmeric, fenugreek, cumin, and chilies, but some include additional spices such as ginger, cloves, nutmeg, coriander, mustard, garlic, fennel, and black pepper.

Here's a quick look at some everyday spices, and their unexpected benefits.

Black pepper

- As soon as you taste black pepper, it stimulates an increase of hydrochloric acid secretion in the stomach, thereby improving digestion, especially of proteins. This is why black pepper has a long folk medicinal reputation as a carminative, or substance that helps prevent gas.
- Black pepper exerts strong anti-bacterial effects.
- The outer layer of black peppercorns stimulates the breakdown of fat cells.
- A phenol in black pepper called piperine is a potent anti-oxidant and anti-inflammatory agent that also enhances people's absorption of a number of vitamins, minerals, antioxidants, and amino acids.
- Some studies have shown that pepper inhibits the growth of solid tumors.

Cardamom

Cardamom, sometimes called Grains of Paradise, is a pungent, aromatic herb first used around the eighth century; it's a native of India. In test-tube studies, cardamom shows stronger activity than vitamin E or vitamin C. This delicious and fragrant seedpod provides antioxidant protection.

Cinnamon

Cinnamon's history as a spice and medicine dates back to ancient Egypt, and it is mentioned in the Bible. This aromatic tree bark also became one of the first commodities traded between the Near East and Europe. Ceylon cinnamon, now grown around the world, is the best variety.

- Cinnamon stimulates insulin receptors and helps increase cells' ability to use glucose. Thus, cinnamon may significantly help people with adult-onset diabetes normalize their blood sugar levels. In fact, less than half a teaspoon per day of cinnamon reduces blood sugar levels in those with adult-onset diabetes. Just 1 gram per day (approximately a quarter to a half teaspoon) yields a 20 percent drop in blood sugar, and reduces cholesterol and triglyceride levels as well. This is tremendously important information for Perricone Promise followers, because one of the keys to stopping the signs of aging on the face and body is the regulation of blood sugar. It appears that simply swizzling a stick of cinnamon in your tea will provide blood-sugar-lowering benefits.
- Cinnamon helps reduce inflammation.
- Cinnamon's essential oils help stop the growth of bacteria and fungi.
- In a test comparing cinnamon with anise, ginger, licorice, mint, nutmeg, vanilla, and the synthetic food preservatives BHA and BHT, cinnamon prevented oxidation more effectively than anything but mint.
- The mere scent of cinnamon enhances the brain's cognitive processing, including attention, memory, and visual–motor speed.
- Cinnamon is prized in ayurvedic and traditional Chinese medicine for its warming qualities, and is used to provide relief from colds or flu. When you feel an infection coming on, try a tea of cinnamon bark and fresh ginger.

Coriander seeds

In the European herbal tradition, coriander was used as an antidiabetic agent; in India's ayurvedic medicine tradition, it is prized for its anti-inflammatory properties. Recent research supports these beliefs, and indicates that coriander can lower levels of total and LDL (bad) cholesterol while increasing levels of HDL (good) cholesterol. Coriander is rich in beneficial phytonutrients, including flavonoids and phenolic acids.

Cumin

Research studies indicate that cumin seeds possess strong antioxidant, anti-inflammatory, anti-cancer, analgesic, and anti-microbial properties. Cumin and cumin oil boost the all-important glutathione levels within the body, increase blood flow, and increase the liver's ability to synthesize important compounds while dramatically improving the flow of bile. Cumin oil has very impressive antiseptic powers, blocks the formation of fungal poisons, and is deadly to parasites, bacteria, and fungi. A recent study reported that black cumin seed essential oil acts as a potent analgesic and anti-inflammatory drug.

Fenugreek

This fibrous seed and curry constituent is a traditional ayurvedic treatment for diabetes and obesity. Research confirms that it stabilizes blood sugar as effectively as the drug glibenclamide, reduces blood lipid levels, and demonstrates strong antioxidant and anti-inflammatory properties in animal models of diabetes. It also has marked anti-cancer and anti-microbial properties.

A recent study found that an amino acid in fenugreek seeds (4-hydroxyisoleucine) can reduce insulin resistance—a marker and early warning sign of diabetes—through activation of the early steps of insulin signaling in peripheral tissues and the liver. In addition, this amino acid improves insulin sensitivity, a very valuable therapeutic effect in diabetes treatment and in an anti-aging regimen. It also possesses anti-glycating abilities—very important in preventing wrinkled skin.

When you think about it, we humans are luckier than many other animal species. We do not have to eat the same foods over and over again. By combining rainbow foods, superfoods, herbs, and spices, we have literally millions of menu choices. We also have ways to supplement our bodies with nutrients we do not, or cannot, get from the foods we eat. In the next chapter, you'll learn about polysaccharides—an exciting new way to boost energy levels from the inside out.

STEP TWO

———

THE SUPPLEMENTS

Boosting Production in Your Energy Factory

The Potent Power of Polysaccharides

I hope I die before I get old.
—THE WHO, "MY GENERATION"

If I had known I was going to live this long, I would have taken better care of myself!
—JAZZ LEGEND EUBIE BLAKE
ON HIS NINETIETH BIRTHDAY

LUCKILY FOR PETE TOWNSHEND, of the band The Who, who penned the memorable words above back in 1965, this pronouncement did not come true! In fact, he and some of his original bandmates (like another band from this era, described below in Rick's Story) are still going strong.

The story of Eubie Blake is even more amazing. Born in 1883, Eubie enjoyed great success in the 1920s as a jazz and ragtime star. Eubie toured USO shows with his band during World War II. He began studying formal music composition in 1946, earning a degree from New York University. Although largely inactive during the 1950s, Eubie made a few appearances in ragtime revivals.

Eubie remained a forgotten unknown until 1969 when, at the age of eighty-six, he recorded a double album called *The Eighty-Six Years of Eubie Blake.* Eubie's popularity soared, and he was much in demand at jazz festivals and concerts. Eubie also lectured at colleges across the country. He formed his own recording company in 1972. Eubie was awarded the Presidential Medal of Freedom in 1981.

Eubie continued to perform until he was ninety-eight years old. He died on February 12, 1983, at the age of one hundred (and five days) in New York City.

Without a crystal ball into the future, we have no idea which direction our lives will take. Will you be performing live at Madison Square Garden on your fifty-ninth birthday to a crowd of adoring fans half your age? Or perhaps, like Eubie, you will be forming your own record company at the age of ninety! Truth is definitely stranger than fiction.

As a physician, I want you to maintain excellent health and vitality regardless of your age. And as a dermatologist I want to make sure that you maintain the radiant, healthy skin of your youth for as long as possible.

That's what the last three food chapters have been about: learning about the foods with the highest antioxidant, anti-inflammatory properties, to help ensure both longevity and vitality.

Improving Fuel Efficiency at the Factory Level

If you're going to improve the quality of the fuel your body produces, you have to start at the source—the "factory" where the food we eat is converted to energy in our bodies. This conversion is accomplished by tiny structures within our cells called mitochondria.

That's why I was so excited when, during the course of my research, I found that scientists at universities in the United States and Asia had discovered a previously unknown class of polysaccharides (chains of linked sugar molecules) that produce dramatic effects on the efficiency and integrity of the mitochondria. This is of great importance because malfunctions in the mitochondria cause many diseases, and also accelerate aging.

Without healthy mitochondria, the body ages rapidly and is highly susceptible to disease. For example, a landmark paper published in 2004 in the highly prestigious scientific journal *Nature* showed that small genetic defects in rodent mitochondria produce all the classic signs of aging. And work by top cell scientists indicates that misfolding of cellular proteins—a malfunction related to mitochondrial health—may cause half or more of all disease conditions, most notably Alzheimer's disease.

The discovery of these important polysaccharides provided me with a new avenue to explore in my quest to find the ideal foods, supplements, and cosmeceuticals to support skin and body health. I began an in-depth study of how these polysaccharides might work together with peptides, neuropeptides, and essential fatty acids (EFAs) to enhance skin and overall health.

This led to the development of a powerful nutritional energy drink rich in all the elements above—a formula I've awarded the appropriate nickname *PEP*.

Add PEP to Your Day and Pump Up Your Cells

What you're doing when you start your day with a teaspoon of Peptide Functional Food (PEP) powder in 6 ounces of water, which is what I recommend in the 28-Day Perricone Program, is improving and increasing the amount of energy produced in your cells. (Don't worry, the PEP formula is not gritty or cloudy like some powdered fiber drinks. It actually has a tasty, slightly nutty flavor.) To create a food that would exert the most powerful possible effects, it is necessary to combine complementary plant food elements. I believe that we can obtain maximum benefits by adding four groups of nutrients:

1. *Lignans from flaxseed hulls.* These healthful, phytoestrogenic fibers possess proven powers to control blood sugar and insulin, and help reduce the risk of diabetes, certain hormone-dependent cancers such as breast and prostate, and cardiovascular disease. Flax lignans also help improve gastrointestinal health, thus enhancing absorption and elimination of foods, and appear to enhance the antioxidant power and energy-generating capacity of the cells' mitochondria.

2. *Amino acids and polypeptides.* The PEP functional food contains all eight essential amino acids needed for making the proteins in our connective tissues (including the skin's collagen and elastin), plus ten

more selected for their beneficial effects on the energy-producing capacity of our cells. They are also needed as raw material for all enzymatic processes, including those that help give collagen strength and elasticity.

3. *Vitamins and minerals.* Selected essential nutrients with particular benefits on the body's antioxidant and tissue-repair systems.

4. *Dietary fibers.* Selected soluble and insoluble fibers to help control blood sugar and enhance digestion.

This combination of nutrients enables you to "pump up" the cells so that they can work at their highest efficiency during the day, when you need them most.

And you'll enjoy a much greater energy boost (and a much healthier one) with the PEP formula than you do with a morning cup of coffee. I doubt that anyone is ever going to walk into the corner coffee shop and order a nice cool "Grande Polysaccharide, please." But if you want that extra energy to start your day, you're much better off with one teaspoon of PEP in eight ounces of water than with sixteen ounces of caffeine-laden coffee. First of all, coffee is acidic and dehydrates your skin. Even worse, drinking coffee has been shown to increase the amounts and effects of the stress hormone cortisol—including lowering blood circulation to the brain, compromising the immune system, and increasing blood pressure and insulin levels. For a healthier start to the day, try a PEP drink followed by a cup of green tea.

The Potent Power of PEP

I consider the PEP formulation a superior *functional food,* which the U.S. Institute of Medicine defines as "those foods that encompass potentially healthful products including any modified food or ingredient that may provide a health benefit beyond the traditional nutrients it contains."

And because it is a food, its effects are physiologic—that is, the PEP formula works with the body to nourish and repair tissues. This means that the body does not need continuous high levels of PEP food to enjoy its benefits over time. In fact, the opposite is true. After the first month or two, intake can be cut in half with ongoing positive results.

These are some of the key benefits of the PEP functional beverage:

- Increased physical and mental energy.
- Increased circulation in the muscles, heart, brain, and other organs.
- More vibrant, soft, supple skin.
- Increased production of antioxidants to help protect against oxidative damage and free-radical attacks on all body cells.
- Reduced inflammation throughout the body.
- Increased production of fibroblasts, the cells that build tissues in the skin and elsewhere.
- Increases in the cells' uptake of glucose, thus reducing hyperinsulinemia (too much insulin) and the common metabolic dysfunction called Syndrome X that leads to inflammation, diabetes, and heart disease.

Rick's Story: Rescuing an Anxious Rock Star

As someone who came of age in the late 1960s, I believe that some of the best popular music was created during these turbulent years. In fact, much of this music is still tremendously popular today, with many groups of the 1960s still touring to sellout crowds. I admit to feeling a bit of a thrill when one of the most famous rock icons of my generation contacted me.

"Dr. Perricone, I need help," Rick (not his real name!) said without preamble. "I have a sold-out tour looming on the horizon and my energy levels are pretty low. Sure, once on stage the adrenaline kicks in"—and no doubt other helpful stimulant substances, I thought to myself—"but I have to get myself ready for all the rest that touring entails," he explained.

Rick spent a lot of his time in the Caribbean, where he had a palatial estate worthy of his world-class rock star status. When he wasn't sitting by the pool, he was out on his sailboat. Consequently, his skin had suffered a significant amount of sun damage. In fact, he had a lot of wrinkles. Although he had dropped many bad habits of his youth, including chain-smoking, Rick was no saint, and the years of life in the fast lane were taking their toll.

Rick was also somewhat of a legend when it came to women and was currently dating a very young model—additional motivation for him to get going on a rejuvenation program.

"So, Doc, what's first?" he asked. "When do I go under the knife?"

"Rick, that is not the answer for you," I said. "We're going to do this the 'natural' way." Since he was also a child of the 1960s, I was hoping that this holistic approach would appeal to him. "First, you have to start with an anti-inflammatory diet and an anti-inflammatory nutritional supplement program, which will be a great help for overall energy and stamina. Then we introduce the fun parts of the rejuvenation process, which include working with some very cool substances known as neuropeptides," I explained. I also planned to have a case of wild Alaskan salmon shipped to Rick, because this is a cornerstone of the anti-inflammatory program. I instructed Rick to eat the salmon four or five times a week—it is incomparable for rejuvenation of both the skin and the brain.

I knew that Rick would be one of the all-time challenges of my career. I needed to make sure that the nutrients in the food and supplements that I recommended would actually be bio-available—that is, be able to be properly digested and absorbed. My plan was to start him on the recently developed PEP functional food, which takes the form of a powdered drink mix.

It was my goal in creating the PEP cell-power drink to have a highly concentrated nutrient substance that would work synergistically with the entire Perricone Promise 28-Day Program to maximize its anti-aging benefits. With the introduction of polysaccharide-based nutrition—such as in the PEP drink formula—we can deliver highly efficient fuel to the cells' mitochondria in a way that is safe, effective, and affordable. Rick was the ideal candidate to prove its efficacy. And he was eager to get started.

Before continuing with Rick's Story, I should explain that the PEP formula works primarily by providing the body with unique polysaccharides called *alpha-glucans,* which help increase the energy in our cells and help the skin repair, renew, and revitalize itself. The vitamins, minerals, and amino acids in the PEP formula benefit the skin directly by helping with the synthesis of structural collagen and elastin, and by protecting it from free radicals and the sun's UV damage. The essential fatty acids nourish the skin, and help keep it hydrated and silky smooth.

In addition to the PEP food, I started Rick on thymic peptide supplements, a Total Skin and Body nutritional supplement program, and topical neuropeptide products. I recommended my three-step neuropeptide program, and suggested that he start with a neuropeptide facial serum prep to totally saturate his skin with a neuropeptide/DMAE combination. This would enable his skin to receive the maximum benefits of a neuropeptide facial conformer. Because Rick had so many wrinkles, I recommended that he do this morning and evening—for most people, once a day application is all that is needed. As a final step, I wanted Rick to liberally massage the Neuropeptide Contour Cream on his face and throat to help counteract the sagging.

Four weeks later I received two tickets to Rick's kick-off concert at Madison Square Garden—as well as a couple of backstage passes. After a quick mental lament on what these tickets would have meant to my popularity a couple of decades ago, I made a note on my calendar to attend.

The day of the concert dawned clear and bright, and as I drove into the city I realized how much I was looking forward to the show. However, nothing quite prepared me for the spectacle that unfolded over the next three hours. Rick and his group performed with the drive and energy of sixteen-year-olds, and the screaming fans kept up an equally impressive performance.

I made my way backstage, hoping it had been the combination of the anti-inflammatory diet and supplements along with the neuropeptides that was responsible for such a transformation in Rick.

> *Although he was a bit tired after the show, I could see immediately that Rick's newfound energy was the result of his past four weeks on the program. His skin glowed, thanks to the increase in healthy circulation delivered by the neuropeptides. His lines and wrinkles appeared to have much less depth, and overall his skin appeared more firm, smooth, and supple.*
>
> *"I really want to thank you, Doc," Rick said, smiling broadly. "This peptide stuff is something else. I feel like a new man."*
>
> *And truth be told, he looked like one, too.*

PEP Versus Syndrome X

Research shows that the PEP functional food I gave Rick has another unexpected benefit: It helps correct an increasingly prevalent cluster of metabolic imbalances called Syndrome X, which is seen in diabetes and obesity as well as cardiovascular disease. The Maitake Fraction-SX formula, which you will read about later in this chapter, is also of major importance in fighting Syndrome X.

Syndrome X is identified by four features:

1. Abdominal obesity (excessive fat tissue in the abdominal region)
2. Glucose intolerance
3. Dyslipidemia (high blood triglyceride levels and low HDL cholesterol levels)
4. High blood pressure

Syndrome X is closely associated with disturbances in glucose–insulin metabolism (also known as insulin resistance; see the sidebar), which the polysaccharide/peptide food improves in several ways:

- Through their effects on the signaling systems in the digestive tract, alpha-glucans enhance the efficiency with which the body produces insulin in response to the sugars and carbohydrates we ingest. (Insulin is required to transport glucose into our cells, where it is "burned" for energy.)

- Syndrome X suppresses the body's production of dehydroepiandrosterone (DHEA)—the precursor hormone to anti-aging hormones such as testosterone, estrogen, and human growth hormone—by as much as 50 percent. Because the nutrients in the PEP food reduce the effects of Syndrome X, they help the body produce as much of the anti-aging hormone DHEA as it needs.

- Alpha-glucans act like dietary fiber to slow the absorption of regular dietary sugars—an effect that further helps to balance the body's sugar–insulin metabolic process.

- The polypeptides in the PEP food provide a superior source of the raw materials needed to manufacture insulin as well as the amino acids critical to the production of anti-aging antioxidants such as glutathione.

INSULIN RESISTANCE

As someone who has devoted decades of research into the causes of aging, I have long been concerned with a condition known as insulin resistance. Insulin is the hormone responsible for getting energy, in the form of glucose (blood sugar), into our cells. Inside the cell, glucose is either used for energy or stored for future use in the form of glycogen in liver or muscle cells. When we are insulin-resistant, insulin levels climb higher and higher, but the blood sugar doesn't get into our cells. This means that high levels of insulin and blood sugar continue to circulate, leading to increased glycation of proteins—and damaged tissues that generate a continuous stream of free radicals, which promote inflammation and aging.

Excess blood insulin also increases the risk of diabetes. About one-third of people with insulin resistance will develop type 2 (adult) diabetes. We are witnessing a virtual diabetes epidemic. The prevalence of diabetes is increasing 4 to 5 percent annually, with an estimated 40 to 45 percent of people over sixty-five years of age at most risk. Many working in the field believe that this percentage will increase even further as baby boomers enter their fifties and sixties.

And a recent study in the *New England Journal of Medicine* found that mitochondria do not appear to function properly in the children of parents with type 2 diabetes. This defect could lead to an accumulation of fat inside muscle cells and to the development of insulin resistance. The real tragedy is that often we could avoid these problems by making healthier food choices, by exercising, and by moderating our high-stress lifestyles. Even if we don't develop diabetes, low-grade insulin resistance can accelerate aging throughout the body, including visible signs such as wrinkles. To make matters worse, insulin resistance becomes more prevalent with advancing age, and worsens many chronic disorders.

The results of diabetes and cardiovascular studies have led the scientists who conducted the studies to hypothesize that the revolutionary polysaccharides in the PEP food formula work with its EFAs, flax lignans, amino acids, vitamins, and minerals to enhance cellular energy, rejuvenation, and repair (see the Resource Guide for information on how to obtain PEP). Major studies are scheduled at research universities to verify that this formulation will produce the clinical benefits seen via the mechanisms hypothesized. I recommend just one small serving per day. This can help deliver optimum nutrition to your cells, thereby conferring a variety of benefits, including youthful, healthy, radiant skin.

Maitake Magic: Mushroom Polysaccharides

Now that I've covered the myriad benefits of the amazing polysaccharides in the PEP beverage mix, I'd like to share information about another source of healthful polysaccharides—those found in fungi, including the mushrooms prominent in traditional Chinese medicine.

I recently spoke to Harry G. Preuss, M.D., MACN, CNS, at Georgetown University School of Medicine, about maitake mushrooms. Dr. Preuss is the highly regarded author of the book *Maitake Magic* as well as coauthor of a number of scientific studies on maitake. According to Dr. Preuss, extracts derived from maitake and other mushrooms are considered front-line medical "drugs" throughout much of the world, even though the scientific study of mushrooms has only begun during the last twenty years.

WHAT'S A MAITAKE?

The maitake (my-*tah*-key) is a large mushroom that grows deep in the mountains of northeastern Japan (where it is known as the "king of the mushrooms") as well as in North America and Europe. It has long been known for its medicinal properties; in fact, it was so prized in feudal Japan that it was exchanged for its weight in silver by local lords, who in turn offered it to the shogun.

Most medicinal mushrooms—such as reishi, shiitake, cordyceps, and maitake—contain polysaccharides called beta-glucans that stimulate cell-mediated immunity. In other words, mushrooms seem to "turn on" cells in the immune system, including macrophages (large cells that can digest foreign substances in the body) and T cells that appear to have significant cancer- and infection-fighting properties.

In addition to immunity benefits, specific beta-glucan fractions (polysaccharide compounds) in the maitake offer additional health benefits, including enhanced control of blood sugar, cholesterol, blood pressure, and body weight. While many fungi can be used as a source of beta-glucans, maitake is substantially different in that it can be taken orally in powder form or made into a liquid that can be injected—and it appears to works equally well either way.

In the 28-Day Perricone Program, you will see that I recommend you start the day with a teaspoon of my PEP formula. As an alternative to that, I suggest you take a maitake supplement every day, choosing from one of the two types below:

- *Fraction-SX.* The beta-glucans in maitake mushrooms have a stabilizing effect on blood sugar and insulin levels. They sensitize the cells to insulin, which makes them an effective weapon in the fight against Syndrome X and insulin resistance.
- *Fraction-D.* Studies have shown that the unique chemical structure of maitake's beta-glucan polysaccharides can actually help shrink the size of some cancer tumors. When mice with melanoma (a lethal form of skin cancer) were injected with the beta-glucan polysaccharides found in maitake mushrooms, their tumor weight decreased by about 70 percent; the beta-glucan also inhibited the spread of the cancer to the lungs. Research on the D-Fraction of maitake indicates that it exerts the strongest cancer inhibition of any dietary source of beta-glucans.

  Bacterial infections also respond to Maitake D-Fraction polysaccharides, as do many viral infections, from the common cold and flu to herpes and HIV. They even mitigate the toxic effects of radiation and chemotherapy while augmenting their cancer-killing effects, resulting in prolonged survival and improved quality of life for cancer patients. For information on where to get maitake mushroom products, see the Resource Guide.

These polysaccharide products may seem strange to you. That's because they're "new"—but new and fascinating facts about how the body works are being discovered every day. And as we live longer and longer lives, the battle against aging has to find newer and better weapons with which we can arm ourselves. In many ways, supplements are technologically advanced weapons to keep ourselves in the best shape possible. In the next chapter, you'll discover more about specific anti-aging, anti-inflammatory, and fat-metabolizing supplements that can help your body maintain maximum efficiency for a long time to come.

7 Adding to a Healthier You

Anti-Aging, Anti-Inflammatory, and Fat-Metabolizing Supplements

I don't want to achieve immortality through my work . . . I want to achieve it through not dying.

—WOODY ALLEN

WHEN YOU FOLLOW THE PERRICONE PROMISE 28-Day Program in chapter 9, you'll be including the rainbow foods, superfoods, and herbs and spices described in the last several chapters and be well on your way to gaining and maintaining the program's healthy benefits. To ratchet those benefits up an additional notch, there are several anti-aging, anti-inflammatory, and fat-burning supplements that can increase your ability to reach optimum appearance and health.

The foods and supplements recommended in *The Perricone Promise* were selected for a number of reasons, including their ability to reduce the negative effects of dietary starches and sugars, provide optimum nutrition, enhance cognitive (thinking) ability, and, last but not least, help keep skin radiant and supple. They also work synergistically with topical antioxidants to help stave off many of the unnecessary ravages of time. If you have read *The Perricone Prescription* or *The Wrinkle Cure,* you know that cornerstones of my supplement program include alpha lipoic acid (ALA), vitamin C ester, and dimethylaminoethanol (DMAE)—all of which I continue to recommend. We all need essential vitamins, minerals, and other nutrients to stay young and healthy. In this chapter, in addition to a complete list of the total skin and body nutrients that I recommend you take every day, I'll briefly review the benefits of some of these old friends, and introduce you to some exciting new anti-aging supplements.

I have selected these supplements from among the many available choices because they offer powerful protection from the effects of inflammation, particularly when caused by dietary starches and sugars.

The supplements have been divided into four areas:

1. *Anti-glycation supplements.*
   Alpha lipoic acid
   Benfotiamine
   Carnosine

2. *Fat metabolizers/energy boosters.*
   Conjugated linoleic acid
   Chromium polynicotinate
   Alpha lipoic acid
   Acetyl-L-carnitine (ACL)
   L-carnitine fumarate
   Essential fatty acids (EFAs)
   CoQ10

3. *Anti-aging/energy boosters/antioxidant/anti-inflammatory.*
   Alpha lipoic acid
   Acetyl-L-carnitine
   CoQ10
   Vitamin C
   Vitamin E
   Essential fatty acids
   DMAE
   Calcium
   Magnesium
   Manganese

4. *Wound healing and wrinkle prevention.*
   Thymic peptides
   Copper

Of course, many of the supplements that are listed in each category also possess significant crossover activity into the other categories.

The following chart presents a snapshot of the properties of each supplement, based primarily on the current research, but also reflecting the results in my patients and myself.

IMPORTANT ANTI-AGING SUPPLEMENTS AND THEIR PROPERTIES						
	ANTI-GLYCATION	ANTI-INFLAMMATORY	ANTI-OXIDANT	FAT BURNING/WEIGHT CONTROL	CELLULAR ENERGY BOOSTER	GENERAL ANTI-AGING BENEFITS
ALPHA-LIPOIC ACID	X	X	X	X	X	Cell protection and cellular energy
ACETYL-CARNITINE	X		X	X	X	Cellular energy, fat metabolizer
BENFOTIAMINE	X	X			X	Anti-glycation
L-CARNITINE				X	X	Cellular energy
CARNOSINE	X	X		X	X	Anti-glycation, cell protein protection
CONJUGATED LINOLEIC ACID (CLA)		X	X	X		Anti-cancer/anti-obesity effects
CoQ10		X	X	X	X	Antioxidant/energy benefits
DMAE		X				Stabilized cell membranes
GAMMA LINOLEIC ACID (GLA)		X				Anti-inflammatory benefits
OMEGA-3 FATTY ACIDS		X		X	X	Brain and heart benefits
VITAMIN C (ESPECIALLY ESTER FORM)		X	X		X	Antioxidant effects
VITAMIN E / TOCOTRIENOLS	X	X	X			Antioxidant, heart, and skin benefits
THYMIC PEPTIDES		X				Nerve and endocrine benefits

The Triple Crown—the Anti-Glycating Agents

If you want to maintain beautiful skin and properly functioning organ systems, start by eliminating the high-glycemic foods that cause sudden spikes in blood sugar (glucose) levels. High-glycemic foods do their damage via a process that proceeds in three silent but deadly steps: They (1) boost blood sugar levels, which (2) increases insulin and inflammation which produces glycation (binding of sugar molecules to proteins), which (3) creates the free-radical factories called advanced glycation end-products (AGEs), all of which further increases cellular inflammation.

As we learned in Brett's Story in chapter 3, when foods rapidly convert to sugar in the bloodstream, as sugar and high-glycemic carbohydrates do, they cause glycation. Glycation can occur in skin as well, creating detrimental age-related changes to collagen—and that means deep wrinkles. When glycation occurs in your skin, the sugar molecules attach themselves to the collagen fibers, where they trigger a series of spontaneous chemical reactions. The end result is the irreversible cross-linking between adjoining collagen molecules and loss of skin elasticity that you learned about in chapter 1.

In fact, glycation and oxidation form a vicious cycle in that glycation can be the result of free-radical damage, and once the proteins are glycated, they continuously generate free radicals. The AGEs I talked about earlier also produce free radicals that specifically activate the pro-inflammatory peptide TNF-a, tissue levels of which are normally elevated in the elderly and in Alzheimer's disease, and which are believed to promote degeneration of the nerves and brain.

The best course of action is prevention, which can be accomplished by avoiding pro-inflammatory sugars and starches. Unfortunately, our brains are programmed to derive pleasure from consuming refined carbohydrates via a sugar- and starch-driven boost in serotonin levels. To make matters worse, these carbs are almost impossible to escape—we are bombarded by their siren songs in restaurants and supermarkets and through print and broadcast advertising. Fortunately, the dangers of these foods are finally beginning to sink into our collective consciousness—and not a minute too soon, because we're facing unprecedented obesity and diabetes epidemics. Our culture has an obsession with staying young, thin, and beautiful by any means possible. The healthiest way to accomplish this, however, is to follow the Perricone Promise, which will help keep your brain functioning efficiently, help keep your energy at optimum levels, and help keep your skin firm and radiant.

For those reasons, it makes sense to begin the fight against glycation with three powerful supplements: benfotiamine, carnosine, and alpha lipoic acid.

BENFOTIAMINE: ANTI-GLYCATING VARIANT OF VITAMIN B$_1$

One of the most exciting new nutritional defenses against the effects of skin- and body-destroying glycation is a fat-soluble, highly absorbable form of vitamin B$_1$ (thiamine) called benfotiamine or benfothiamine. Benfotiamine was developed in Japan in the late 1950s to treat neuropathy (nerve damage) in alcoholics, as well as to treat sciatica and other painful nerve conditions.

Benfotiamine is a synthetic derivative of vitamin B$_1$ that shows promise in treating a number of neurological and vascular conditions. It also appears to have beneficial anti-aging qualities, protecting human cells from harmful metabolic end-products.

Benfotiamine is one of the most effective anti-glycating nutrients available because it blocks three of the major biochemical pathways through which hyperglycemia (high blood sugar) does its pro–inflammatory damage, including the formation of AGEs.

In addition to blocking inflammatory pathways, benfotiamine also enhances the activity of an enzyme called transketolase, which (like alpha lipoic acid) prevents activation of the pro-inflammatory cellular compound NF-kappa B. It also converts harmful blood sugar metabolites (glucose breakdown products) into harmless chemicals.

While standard water-soluable vitamin B$_1$ also works to blunt the damage caused by high blood sugar levels, fat-soluble benfotiamine exerts more powerful effects, using smaller doses. Benfotiamine can also be found in one of our Ten Superfoods (see chapter 4), foods in the Allium family (garlic, onions, shallots, and leeks)—another health benefit of these easy-to-find, easy-to-use pungent vegetables.

Benfotiamine is also a very safe supplement. Standard thiamine (vitamin B_1) shows no adverse effects even at high doses (several hundred milligrams a day), and safety tests indicate that benfotiamine is even safer.

To learn more about benfotiamine, read the studies, order the products, and/or go to these Web sites: www.nvperriconemd.com, www.benfotiamine.org, and www.benfotiamine.net.

**U.S. Recommended Daily Intake (RDI): None established.
**Perricone Promise Recommendation: 300 mg per day (150 mg at breakfast and dinner).

CARNOSINE (B-ALANYL-L-HISTIDINE)

Carnosine is a naturally occurring dipeptide found in high concentrations in our brains, our muscle tissues, and the lens of the eye. A 2001 study by Professor John W. Baynes, Ph.D., a leading glycation researcher, revealed that carnosine and all other known glycation inhibitors—such as the prescription drug aminoguanidine—work in large part by chelating (binding to) copper in the body. (Research shows that copper in our bodies, while essential in small amounts, also stimulates oxidation and glycation.)

Carnosine is also a very special kind of antioxidant. While many antioxidants can help protect our cells from free radicals, carnosine has the rare ability to repair or remove damaged or "misfolded" proteins. This misfolding occurs normally in our cells and is increased when our nutrition, hygiene, or lifestyle becomes compromised. Experts in protein function believe that the misfolding of proteins may account for as much as half of all human disease, directly or indirectly. (Alzheimer's and mad cow are only the most famous examples of diseases linked to protein damage.) Carnosine's amazing list of anti-aging effects on the brain reinforces the concepts behind the Brain–Beauty Connection.

These are just some of carnosine's beneficial anti-aging effects:

- Protects the cellular antioxidants superoxide dismutase (SOD) and catalase, cellular DNA, and key molecules—including amyloid beta—from glycation. (Glycated amyloid beta constitutes the brain tissue "plaque" believed to cause or promote Alzheimer's disease.)
- Binds to excess copper-zinc in the brain. (Copper-zinc chelators dissolve Alzheimer's disease plaques.)
- Protects against excitotoxicity—the damaging overactivity of the neurotransmitter glutamate that is largely responsible for the devastating effects of brain plaque in Alzheimer's disease, as well as the death of brain and nerve cells.
- Prevents damaged proteins from damaging healthy proteins; helps recycle damaged proteins.
- Enhances and balances immune functions and nerve transmission.
- Speeds wound healing and recovery from muscle fatigue.
- Helps lower blood pressure, thereby reducing stress and hyperactivity and promoting sleep.
- Protects nerve cells (neurons) from damage and death, making it a promising treatment for patients with stroke.

**U.S. Recommended Daily Intake (RDI): None established.
**Perricone Promise Recommendation: 250 to 1,000 mg per day, in divided dosages. There is some controversy about the most effective dosage, with scientists arguing for both the lower end and higher end of the dose.

ALPHA LIPOIC ACID

Here's an idea of the power of this "universal antioxidant": It is four hundred times more effective than both vitamin C and E combined. ALA actually helps curtail glycation and enhances the transfer of blood sugar into the cells by stimulating glucose uptake. (I will address ALA in more depth under Anti-Aging All-Stars later in this chapter.)

**U.S. Recommended Daily Intake (RDI): None established.
**Perricone Promise Recommendation: 200 mg per day, in two doses of 100 mg at breakfast and dinner.

Fat Metabolizers/Energy Boosters

CLA (conjugated linoleic acid) and chromium polynicotinate show great promise as supplements that exert a positive effect on body composition.

CLA: A PROMISING FAT-MELTER AND MORE

While certain nutrients are involved in the metabolism of fat—including carnitine, chromium, and essential fatty acids—none of these cell-level metabolic factors has shown significant positive effects in clinical trials of weight control.

A few years ago, however, university scientists researching fatty components of milk fat found one type with the promising potential to improve body composition while reducing the risk of diabetes and certain cancers. This once obscure nutrient—a group of related linoleic acid isomers collectively called conjugated linoleic acid, found in red meats, poultry, and dairy foods—has since been sub-jected to several well-controlled clinical trials. Most of the studies in overweight people produced substantial shifts from fat to muscle—changes unequaled by any other weight control supplement.

The positive effects of CLA on body composition have been shown in numerous animal studies, and in most human studies conducted to date. While people in most of the successful trials did not lose weight, they experienced a shift of up to 9 percent from fat to muscle, without making any other dietary changes. No one is sure how CLA works to enhance body composition, but it may balance peptides and prostaglandins, which could optimize muscle growth and fat loss. Other researchers believe that CLA is directly involved in fat metabo-lism, and helps the body burn stored fat. Another theory posits that CLA counteracts the negative effects of corticosteroids such as cortisol, which break down muscle protein and promote fat gain.

CLA has also shown potent anti-diabetes and anti-cancer effects. Its anti-cancer properties may be due to an antioxidant effect or to an interaction between CLA and certain carcinogens. In several studies, CLA normalized blood-sugar-control mechanisms in prediabetic aninals. The effects of CLA in this regard are significant enough that one team concluded, "CLA effects on glucose tolerance and glucose homeostasis indicate that dietary CLA may prove to be an important therapy for the prevention and treatment of NIDDM [adult diabetes]." In a subsequent placebo-controlled clinical trial, adult diabetics who took supplemental CLA for eight weeks reduced their blood sugar levels, reduced their blood levels of leptin—a hormone associated with weight gain—and lost weight.

★★U.S. Recommended Daily Intake (RDI): None established.
★★Perricone Promise Recommendation: 1,000 mg, three to four times per day. Because different forms of CLA produce different effects, it is important to choose CLA supplements that contain "mixed isomers." (See the Resource Guide for my recommendation.) Note to vegetarians: Supplemental CLA is made from vegetable oil.

CHROMIUM POLYNICOTINATE

In human studies, chromium has been found to decrease body fat and enhance lean body mass, while maintaining healthy cholesterol levels already in normal range. In addition, chromium helps maintain a healthy blood sugar level.

★★U.S. Recommended Daily Intake (RDI): 120 mcg.
★★Perricone Promise Recommendation: 200 mcg.

ADDITIONAL SUPPLEMENTS

There are several other supplements that act as fat metabolizers and cellular energy boosters. I have had excellent success in helping patients lose excess weight by adding the following supplements to their daily regimen:

- ALA (alpha lipoic acid): 250 to 500 mg per day.
- CoQ10: 60 to 120 mg per day.
- Acetyl-L-carnitine: 500 to 1,000 mg per day (take on empty stomach).
- L-carnitine: 500 mg, three times per day.
- DMAE: 75 mg, twice per day.

- L-tyrosine: 500 mg, twice per day.
- Gamma linoleic acid: 1,000 mg per day.
- Omega-3 in the form of fish oil containing DHA and EPA: 100 to 150 mg, two or three times per day.
- Omega 6: 750 mg, twice per day.

Anti-Aging All-Stars

The following supplements have proven to be indispensable to an anti-aging program that really works!

ALPHA LIPOIC ACID

In addition to preventing glycation, alpha lipoic acid plays a central role in the body's antioxidant defense network, cellular energy production, and the prevention and repair of collagen damage. Here are just some of its anti-aging benefits:

- ALA is critical at several points in the *Krebs cycle*—a process that provides continuous energy to the cell. Free radicals are produced as a by-product of the Krebs cycle, but ALA (like CoQ10) helps neutralize them.
- ALA is an extraordinarily broad-spectrum antioxidant, able to quench a wide range of free radicals in both the aqueous (water) and lipid (fat) portions of the cell. Moreover, ALA has the remarkable ability to recycle several other important antioxidants, including vitamins C and E, glutathione, and CoQ10.
- ALA is also the only antioxidant that can boost cellular levels of glutathione, the tripeptide antioxidant of tremendous importance in overall health and longevity. Besides being the body's primary water-soluble antioxidant and a major detoxification agent, glutathione is essential for the functioning of the immune system. People with chronic illnesses such as AIDS, cancer, and autoimmune diseases generally have very low levels of glutathione. White blood cells are particularly sensitive to changes

in glutathione levels, and even subtle changes may have profound effects on the immune response.

- ALA also exerts several beneficial effects in the prevention and treatment of diabetes. ALA is needed to convert dietary carbohydrates to energy in the cells' mitochondria.

- Last, but far from least, ALA puts the brakes on potentially proinflammatory metabolic factors called nuclear transcription factors (NTFs): specifically, activator protein 1 and nuclear factor kappa B. As people age, cumulative damage by free radicals makes it easier for free radicals to kick NTFs into pro-inflammatory mode. This results in weakened immunity and promotes cancer and various degenerative diseases. ALA helps control inflammation by preventing NTFs from going into the pro-inflammatory mode.

**U.S. Recommended Daily Intake (RDI): None established.
**Perricone Promise Recommendation: 200 mg per day, in two doses of 100 mg at breakfast and dinner.

ACETYL-L-CARNITINE

Acetyl-L-carnitine is central to the production of cellular energy. ACL also improves energy production within brain cells, and is considered a neuroprotective agent because of its antioxidant and membrane-stabilizing effects. Acetyl-L-carnitine differs from L-carnitine in that it can pass through the blood–brain barrier and therefore help rejuvenate brain cells more efficiently than L-carnitine. My recommendation is to take both acetyl-L-carnitine and L-carnitine daily.

This overlooked nutritional factor, which is present in beef, pork, and chicken, also boosts tissue levels of CoQ10 and glutathione. In addition, ACL restores cortisol receptors and thereby protects nerve cells against the ravages of stress. We all know that stress is one of the primary causes of brain aging—and of wrinkled, sagging skin.

**U.S. Recommended Daily Intake (RDI): None established.
**Perricone Promise Recommendation: 500 mg acetyl-L-carnitine per day, plus 500 mg L-carnitine fumarate three times per day.

COENZYME Q10 (COQ10, UBIQUINONE)

The antioxidant called coenzyme Q10 performs two vital functions: It transports electrons in energy production and protects cells against the free radicals formed during normal metabolism. Thus, CoQ10 protects against the high free-radical activity found in our mitochondria, and is critical to proper functioning of their ability to generate energy. The heart, brain, and muscles appear most affected by age-related declines in CoQ10 levels; studies have shown that coenzyme Q10 supplementation has extended the life spans of mice.

Recent studies indicate that CoQ10 interrupts the chemical chain reaction that transforms essential fatty acids into free radicals. It also reduces blood levels of lipid peroxides (key markers of overall oxidative stress in the body), and boosts blood levels of the antioxidant vitamins E and C.

★★U.S. Recommended Daily Intake (RDI): None established.
★★Perricone Promise Recommendation: 100 mg per day. (Intakes of 100 to 200 mg per day have been studied with no apparent adverse side effects.) Coenzyme Q10 requires fat for optimum absorption into the bloodstream, so take it with fatty foods, or with essential fatty acid supplements. I recommend the CoQ10 that is formulated specifically to disperse in a water-soluble environment to provide higher serum levels and higher therapeutic benefit. See the Resource Guide for recommendations.

VITAMIN C ESTER: A SUPERIOR "C"

Without vitamin C, people cannot thrive or even survive. While most animals can produce their own vitamin C, humans, primates (apes, monkeys, lemurs), and guinea pigs have lost this ability. This makes it essential to eat foods rich in vitamin C, and take vitamin C supplements as insurance.

Vitamin C (ascorbic acid) is also valuable because it is vital to the production of healthy collagen, helps protect the fat-soluble vitamins A and E as well as fatty acids from oxidation, and reduces inflammation throughout the body.

Certain areas of the brain—especially the *nucleus accumbens* (vital to movement control) and *hippocampus* (vital to memory)—contain very high concentrations of vitamin C, which decline as we age. When accompanied by decreases in glutathione, the body becomes swamped with oxidizing free radicals, and oxidation-damaged fats (lipids) accumulate in our cells and tissues.

The "regular" vitamin C (ascorbic acid) found in foods and almost all supplements is water soluble, and cannot protect cell membranes or maintain adequate skin levels in the face of oxidative stress from internal sources and sunlight. (Ascorbic acid also rapidly degrades in most topical skin care products.)

Fortunately, there is another form of vitamin C called ascorbyl palmitate, or vitamin C ester (which consists of ascorbic acid molecules joined to a fatty acid from palm oil), that realizes this essential nutrient's full potential as an anti-aging agent; it exerts greater activity in human cells than ascorbic acid does—and at lower doses. Because ascorbyl palmitate can reside in the fatty cell membrane, it continuously regenerates the vitamin E depleted by that fat-soluble antioxidant's ongoing fight against free radicals. Ascorbyl palmitate also possesses superior ability to stimulate growth of the cells (fibroblasts) that help produce collagen and elastin in human skin. Vitamin C ester truly is the better vitamin C.

Note: Do not confuse vitamin C ester (ascorbyl palmitate) with the patented "mineral ascorbate" vitamin C product called Ester C, which is not fat soluble and has never been shown to offer any significant advantages over regular vitamin C. In topical preparations, look for vitamin C ester and not ascorbic acid. As a supplement, I recommend both forms of vitamin C to give complete protection to the cell.

**U.S. Recommended Daily Intake (RDI): 60 mg.
**Perricone Promise Recommendation: 1,000 mg vitamin C (as ascorbic acid) and 500 mg vitamin C ester (ascorbyl palmitate).

VITAMIN E WITH TOCOTRIENOLS: ANTI-INFLAMMATORY/ANTIOXIDANT

Unlike all other vitamins, which consist of just one molecule, vitamin E is made up of eight separate phenolic compounds—four tocopherols and four tocotrienols. Of these eight naturally occurring forms of vitamin E, only alpha-tocopherol is found in human blood, which indicates that it is probably the most important member of the vitamin E family to human survival, and explains why it is the only vitamin E compound found in most supplements. However, mixed tocopherols with tocotrienols have proved to be superior supplements.

Vitamin E is the major antioxidant that protects fatty tissues from damage by free radicals. Therefore, its importance to protecting delicate cell membranes and curbing inflammation at the cellular level cannot be overstated.

Vitamin E is an important part of my topical anti-aging program because it provides the skin with powerful protection from the adverse effects of sunlight, and the resulting oxidative stress. The tocotrienols in vitamin E have a particular affinity for skin, offering superior protection against sunlight and other environmental stressors.

**U.S. Recommended Daily Intake (RDI): 30 IU.
**Perricone Promise Recommendation: 400 to 800 IU vitamin E containing mixed tocopherols and tocotrienols.

ESSENTIAL FATTY ACIDS: OMEGA-3S AND GLA

Of the two dozen fats essential to human health, only two cannot be made by your body and must be obtained from foods. Accordingly, these two nutrients are called essential fatty acids. Omega-6 EFA, called linoleic acid (LA), is abundant in cooking oils. The other, linolenic acid (LNA), is an omega-3 EFA. Among their many functions, each type of EFA is critical to immunity, brain function, and the structure and integrity of cell membranes. Cell membranes are a key part of the body's defense system, and increased permeability—which can result from a diet deficient in EFAs—can have devastating effects, allowing free radicals and toxins a passageway into the cell, where they can wreak the kinds of havoc that weaken immunity and accelerate aging. The stiffening of the cell membrane results in decreased flexibility, which reduces nutrient intake and also desensitizes important hormone receptors for insulin and other hormones.

EFAs also nourish the skin, hair, mucous membranes, nerves, and glands, and help prevent cardiovascular disease. The polysaccharide peptide food that I recommend owes its wonderful skin-beautifying power to the fact that it is a very rich and very bio-available form of these essential fatty acids. Fatty acids are the major building blocks of the fats in human bodies and foods, and important sources of energy.

EFAs are also the precursors to the hormone-like compounds prostaglandins, which regulate many body functions on a moment-to-moment basis. They govern blood pressure, the tone of smooth (involuntary) muscles in the blood vessels, and the "stickiness" of blood platelets. EFAs also carry the high energy required by our most active tissues, and are growth enhancing. At intake levels above 12 to 15 percent of total calories, they increase the metabolic rate—an effect that causes the body to burn more fat, resulting in loss of excess weight.

Omega-3 EFAs

Unfortunately, when it comes to EFAs, the American diet is woefully unbalanced: too high in omega-6 EFAs and too low in omega-3 EFAs. Over the last century, the ratio of omega-6 to omega-3 fatty acids in our diet has changed from the estimated prehistoric ratio of 3:1 or 5:1 (the same as the ratio found in human cells) to an alarmingly imbalanced ratio of about 15:1. This sets the stage for increases in the tendency of blood to clot, narrowing of blood vessels and raising of blood pressure, and chronic inflammation. Even the U.S. government recently recommended that Americans consume more omega-3 EFAs.

The best food sources of omega-3 EFAs are fatty fish such as salmon and mackerel. Fish oil is also the best source of omega-3 EFAs because it contains the two types of omega-3 fats—EPA and DHA—that the body can use without modification. (Human breast milk is very rich in omega-3 DHA, which is critical to the formation of healthy brains in infants.)

This is why I am such a strong advocate of wild as opposed to farm-raised Alaskan salmon, a superior source of EPA and DHA, whose ratio of omega-3 to omega-6 EFAs is close to the nutritional ideal, and better than the ratio found in most farm-raised salmon. Significant amounts of omega-3 also occur in nuts, seeds (especially flax), and dark green leafy vegetables.

**U.S. Recommended Daily Intake (RDI): None established.
**Perricone Promise Recommendation: Even if you eat fatty fish several times per week, I recommend fish oil supplements to ensure that you receive enough DHA—a fraction of omega-3 that is important for cardiovascular and brain enhancement. I recommend 2 to 4 fish oil capsules (see the Resource Guide) a day with approximately 250 mg DHA and 150 mg EPA.

Gamma-Linoleic Acid

GLA is one omega-6 EFA that is positively beneficial. It is not found in foods—except borage seed, black currant, and primrose seed oils. Under normal circumstances, the body makes all the GLA it requires from linoleic acid; however, we become deficient in GLA when large amounts of sugar, trans-fatty acids (margarine, hydrogenated oils), red meats, and dairy are consumed. That is why, given the strong anti-inflammatory effects of GLA, I recommend taking supplemental amounts.

**U.S. Recommended Daily Intake (RDI): None established.
**Perricone Promise Recommendation: 250 to 1,000 mg.

DMAE

DMAE, or dimethylaminoethanol, is a nutritional substance with powerful anti-inflammatory properties that is found in fish including wild Alaskan salmon, anchovies, and sardines. In addition to its anti-inflammatory activities, DMAE is important in the production of neurotransmitters, especially the neurotransmitter acetylcholine, which is essential in the communication from one nerve to another and between nerves and muscles. In order for your muscles to contract, the message must be sent from your nerves to your muscles via acetylcholine.

Taking DMAE as a supplement has been shown to increase cognitive function by improving memory and problem-solving ability. It has been shown to assist improvement in such disorders as attention deficit disorder (ADD). DMAE can also have an effect on muscle tone, which can be increased by the additional synthesis of acetyl-choline derived from DMAE. This is very exciting because it gives us a way to actually improve our appearance by counteracting the sag-ging associated with aging.

**U.S. Recommended Daily Intake (RDI): None established.
** Perricone Promise Recommendation: 50 to 100 mg per day.

CALCIUM AND MAGNESIUM: A MARRIAGE MADE IN NUTRITIONAL HEAVEN

No discussion of anti-aging supplements would be complete without these familiar essential minerals, which are important for many rea-sons beyond their well-known role in the formation and protection of healthy bones and teeth. In fact, they are essential in helping to control cellular inflammation; no anti-aging nutritional program would be complete without them. Unfortunately, today's diets tend to be low in magnesium and calcium but high in fructose, a sugar that disrupts the balance of calcium, magnesium, phosphorus, and other minerals in the body. Let's take a closer look at this inseparable couple, whose interactions are vital to healthy bones, nerves, and more.

Calcium

Calcium is best known for its role in maintaining the strength and density of bones. It's also essential to many physical functions, including regulation of inflammation, blood clotting, nerve conduc-tion, muscle contraction, enzyme activity, and cell membrane func-tion. Because these processes are essential to health, the body tries to closely control the amount of calcium in the blood. If dietary intake of calcium is too low, the body will draw on calcium stores in the bones to maintain normal blood concentrations, which eventually leads to osteoporosis.

Your mother probably told you to drink milk for strong bones, but other foods—or supplements—will also do the trick. I strongly rec-ommend calcium supplementation at all ages, especially in teen years and as you grow older. Calcium should be taken with vitamin D and magnesium to be fully useful, and a debate continues over the best form of calcium to take. "Chelated" forms such as calcium citrate, aspartate, or maleate are absorbed by the body a bit better, but are usually costlier than calcium carbonate—the standard supplemental form. Calcium carbonate is a good choice unless your digestive system is weak. If it is, take a chelated version, or increase your calcium carbonate intake to account for the lowered absorption level.

Noninflammatory food sources include yogurt and kefir, sardines or salmon (canned with bones), spinach, cooking greens (collards, kale, turnip), sea vegetables (dulse, kelp, and so on), tofu, nuts, and seeds.

**U.S. Recommended Daily Intake (RDI): 1,000 mg.
**Perricone Promise Recommendation: 1,200 mg per day.

Magnesium

The roles magnesium plays in human health are so diverse that virtually every body system—cardiovascular, digestive, neuroendocrine, and brain—needs it to function properly, as do our muscles, kidneys, and livers. Magnesium supplements can help increase memory and learning, attention span, and resistance to stress.

Magnesium also supports bone strength, and is stored on the surface of our bones as a repository the body can use in case of a dietary deficiency. Unfortunately, the average modern diet offers little magnesium, and most Americans are moderately magnesium-deficient. The average woman gets about 200 mg daily, but the RDI is 300 to 400 mg per day, and some physicians—myself included—recommend 500 mg per day.

Magnesium and calcium work together to help regulate nerve and muscle tone. Magnesium also serves as a "gate blocker" in many nerve cells, to keep out excess calcium and thereby keep nerves relaxed. This explains why magnesium deficiency can trigger muscle tension, soreness, spasms, cramps, and fatigue. Also, some forms of energy cannot be stored in our muscle cells unless adequate supplies of magnesium are available. Because of its effects on the heart muscle, magnesium deficiency can result in arrhythmia, irregular contraction, and increased heart rate.

Finally, hundreds of enzymes that speed up chemical reactions in the body require magnesium in order to help metabolize proteins, carbohydrates, and fats, and allow genes to function properly.

**U.S. Recommended Daily Intake (RDI): 400 mg.
**Perricone Promise Recommendation: Anywhere from half the daily dose of calcium to an equivalent amount: 600 to 1,200 mg per day.

MANGANESE

Manganese performs myriad functions, including hundreds of enzymatic reactions. For the purposes of anti-aging, manganese is most important as an essential component of manganese-dependent superoxide dismutase (MnSOD), which battles damaging free radicals that attack the mitochondria. In fact, this key antioxidant enzyme is found only inside the mitochondria.

Interestingly, the best sources of manganese are the rainbow foods discussed in chapter 3 (especially spinach, cooking greens, and berries); the superfoods addressed in chapter 4 (especially beans, garlic, onions, leeks, seeds, nuts, and buckwheat); and the spices covered in chapter 5 (especially cloves, cinnamon, thyme, pepper, oregano, and mint).

**U.S. Recommended Daily Intake (RDI): None established.
**Perricone Promise Recommendation: 5 mg per day. (Manganese supplementation of 3 to 5 mg per day may cause severe low blood sugar in people with insulin-dependent diabetes, who should consult their doctor before taking it.)

Wrinkles Are Tiny Wounds: Nutritional Skin Repair

When we consider the fact that, in essence, a wrinkle can be considered a wound in the skin, we again turn to the miracle of thymic peptides for their unparalleled ability to assist in wound healing.

THYMIC PEPTIDES

Thymic peptides work by stimulating collagen and elastin. This enables the lower portion of the skin, known as the dermis, to refashion or remodel itself. The research done with the thymic peptides inspired me to formulate a special thymic peptide supplement to add to the daily nutritional supplement regimen as an excellent tool for healing and rejuvenating the skin from the inside out. Ideally, repair will come from taking the thymic peptide supplement in conjunction with regular topical application—a subject I will cover in depth in the next chapter.

We now know that the skin has receptors for many thymic peptides; therefore we know that by combining the right peptides at therapeutic levels in both a supplement and a topical therapy, we can affect the skin in a positive manner in such diverse ways as:

- Increased elastin production.
- Increased collagen production resulting in skin remodeling.
- Decreased inflammation.
- Increased blood vessel growth to help nourish the skin.
- Release of growth hormone and growth factors into the skin, resulting in the production and repair of skin cells.

The peptide supplement that I have developed is not something you need to take every day. During the first two weeks of the 28-Day Plan, I recommend that you take one tablet with breakfast and one at lunch. After two weeks, you can reduce the dosage to one daily, or one every other day.

ADDITIONAL ALLIES IN WOUND HEALING

As a dermatologist, I know that any injury to the skin requires adequate body levels of specific vitamins, minerals, and protein. Vitamins B_5 and C, copper, zinc, magnesium, and manganese are the principal nutrients needed to repair any type of tissue damage, from serious wounds to unwanted wrinkles.

Vitamins play their own part in skin and wound repair, but also control the minerals involved. For example, iron is detrimental to wound healing, and vitamins B_5 (pantothene) and C decrease iron levels at the site of a wound. Copper, magnesium, and manganese enhance wound repair. Vitamins B_5 and C increase the levels of these minerals where needed. Vitamin B_5 greatly speeds repair, increases the number of repair cells, and increases the distance they can travel. Later, vitamin C steps in and works with copper to create strong collagen.

Copper is very important in wound repair, because it creates proper cross-links in the collagen and elastin (elements that give the body structure, such as bone, tendon, and skin) that give these connective tissue proteins resiliency and strength. The body also needs copper to make an important antioxidant known as copper-zinc superoxide dismutase, which is key to proper wound healing. In particular, SOD encourages new tissue to grow, enhances collagen production, and reduces swelling, to heal wounds more effectively and rapidly.

In the early stages of an injury, immune cells rush to the site and emit free radicals to disable invading bacteria and dissolve dead and injured tissue. These free radicals must be neutralized once their work is done, lest they go on to damage the body's own cells. This is where SOD and other antioxidants come in. They regulate free-radical reactions created by immune cells, and promote the repair process. As a result, injuries can use up a majority of the body's supplies of SOD, vitamins C and E, and other antioxidants, so it is important to restore them by consuming the right foods and supplements.

Make sure that your nutritional program includes these important vitamins and minerals as well as adequate protein. This will help prevent additional damage to the skin and organ systems as you age and to help reverse any damage that may already have taken place. In chapter 8, I'll take an in-depth look at how novel topical neuropeptide therapies, containing as many as forty diverse and targeted peptides, are rejuvenating and repairing skin with unprecedented success.

STEP THREE

———

THE TOPICALS

Neuropeptides and the Skin

The "Information Superhighway" Road to Rejuvenation

*The difference between the right word and the almost right word
is the difference between lightning and a lightning bug.*
— MARK TWAIN

*It is confidence in our bodies, minds and spirits that allows us to
keep looking for new adventures, new directions to grow in, and
new lessons to learn—which is what life is all about.*
— OPRAH WINFREY, OPRAH MAGAZINE, MAY 2004

AS MARK TWAIN SO SUCCINCTLY IMPLIED—there is a vast difference between lightning and a lightning bug. To me, the next generation of topical therapies utilizing multiple neuropeptides (the lightning) makes a similar quantum leap when compared to much of the existing topical treatments (the lightning bugs) on the market today.

Up to this point in the book, we've been concentrating on maintaining a healthy body and appearance working from the inside out. That's how it should be, because that's where the problem-causing inflammation starts. But that doesn't mean you can neglect your outside and expect the insides to do all the work. After all, your skin is your most exposed organ. Every day, it's subjected to abuse by every passing particle of dust and dirt, by secondhand smoke, traffic fumes, toxic chemicals, and the harmful rays of the sun.

If you want to look and feel as young as you possibly can for as long as you possibly can, you need to begin with the quality of the food you eat and end with the quality of the products you put on your skin.

159

In this chapter, you'll learn about two important breakthroughs in topical skin care that you'll want to use if you want to:

- Maintain that fresh, rosy look of youth and health.
- Revive dull, lifeless skin.
- Minimize skin discoloration and redness.
- Reduce puffiness around the eyes.
- Reduce dark circles under the eyes.
- Decrease the appearance of fine lines and wrinkles.
- Protect the skin from free-radical damage.
- Decrease sagging and loss of tone.

Ariel's Story

On a recent trip to Los Angeles I ran into Ariel, a former neighbor of mine who had relocated to California.

"Dr. Perricone, this is perfect timing! I am seriously considering a few major surgical procedures and would welcome your guidance," Ariel confided. Although only in her early forties, Ariel showed many signs of aging on her face and neck. "I want to start with a laser resurfacing to see if I can even out my skin tone and erase some of these fine lines in my eye area," she continued. "After that I want to try Botox for the forehead frown lines."

Ariel has the peaches-and-cream complexion prevalent in many blonds and redheads. However, whatever her beauty routine was— or wasn't—her complexion was red and irritated. Her skin appeared dry and lacked radiance. I suspected that Ariel was on a very low-fat, low-protein diet. Not only was she extremely thin, but also her face had lost the youthful contours that only a healthy layer of subcutaneous fat can provide. In addition, the skin on her chin and around her mouth was taking on a wrinkled appearance that made her look older than her years.

I explained to Ariel that I had helped many of my patients diminish fine lines, uneven skin tone, and many other problems usually associated with aging—but it was not through chemical or invasive procedures. I suggested that before she tried these more drastic measures, she give my three-tiered approach a try for three days. If she was happy with the results, I would encourage her to start the 28-Day Program.

I often ask my patients concerned with aging, health, and beauty the following question:

Q: What do a child, someone on the three-day nutritional face-lift, and someone in love all have in common?

A: They all have that special glow that comes from the regulation of neuropeptides.

Certain neuropeptides control blood flow, giving us that rosy glow that children and people in love manifest so beautifully. When we are sick, poorly nourished, dehydrated, or depressed, our complexions become sallow, dull, and gray.

While I can't promise that the Perricone Program will help you fall in love, I can promise that you will re-create that special glow— a glow that everyone will notice.

I explained to Ariel that radiant beauty has to come from the inside—starting with diet. The right foods can help us regulate neuropeptide production and reduce inflammation. This is important because as we age, the production of important neuropeptides, as well as hormones, neurotransmitters, and cell turnover, diminishes while inflammatory chemicals increase.

By following the rainbow foods principle and the 28-Day Program, Ariel would be eating wild Alaskan salmon—a brain food whose nutrients work intensely in the skin, increasing radiance and tone. She would be eating liberal amounts of deeply colored fruits and vegetables, including cantaloupe and blueberries. She would be drinking plenty of water and having two salads a day dressed with olive oil and lemon juice. She would also enjoy snacking on raw, unsalted nuts, such as walnuts and almonds. And she would kick her coffee habit.

I could see Ariel cringe at the idea of eating nuts (aren't they high in fat?) and olive oil (what about my "diet" dressing?).

The right fats plump up the skin—without them, you will age prematurely, and the first place this aging will be visible will be in the face. I explained to Ariel that a bagel, low-fat muffin, or the *ubiquitous rice cake would not only accelerate aging but actually block the body from burning fat. I also pointed out the area around her mouth and chin that had developed a "crepey" appearance.*

"Ariel, with the right foods, nutritional supplements, and a couple of targeted topical formulations, I think we can firm this skin up. Are you willing to give my plan a try?"

I gave Ariel a box of supplements that contained all the necessary nutrients divided into individual packets for ease of use. I also started her on my recently formulated peptide supplement, as well as the PEP functional food with instructions to take one heaping teaspoon mixed with warm water upon arising. Both the peptide supplement and the peptide food have been developed to work synergistically with the most exciting new topical treatments I have come across in more than two decades of research—topical neuropeptide therapy.

Because we had some serious rejuvenation to accomplish for Ariel, I gave her three products. After cleansing with an anti-inflammatory cleanser, Ariel was to apply to her face and throat a peptide serum prep—a clear liquid that would thoroughly saturate the skin with a mixture of peptides and dimethylaminoethanol (DMAE, another anti-inflammatory). Step two was the application of a special peptide facial conformer. The third and final step was the application of a peptide contour cream. This last step was crucial for Ariel, because we needed to lift and firm the throat area and tone and tighten the area around the mouth and chin.

Ariel was a prime candidate for the incomparable power of the topical neuropeptide formulation.

Back to the Brain–Beauty Connection

As you remember from chapter 1, neuropeptides are tiny strings of amino acids found naturally in our bodies that act as messengers controlling many biological functions. Neuropeptides have activity in the brain; however, they also work intensely in the skin. This is because when we are in the embryonic stage of development, the layers of cells that are responsible for making up the brain eventually develop into skin as well. In fact, there is a direct link between the brain and the action of nerves in the skin—thus the Brain–Beauty Connection.

To put it simply, what is therapeutic and active in the brain is also therapeutic and active in the skin.

These natural and nontoxic neuropeptides play important roles in the beauty and appearance of the skin. As we age, the levels of natural neuropeptides, produced by the body, diminish. We have two ways of replenishing and strengthening the neuropeptides in our bodies: through the foods we eat, and now, through applying natural neuropeptides to our skin daily to retain a youthful appearance and slow the signs of premature aging.

Ariel embraced the Perricone Promise wholeheartedly. She admitted to me later that she felt she was at a crossroads. If she didn't do something now to try to regain a more youthful and healthy appearance, it would be all downhill.

"Dr. Perricone, let me tell you, I ate lots of salmon and really enjoyed it!" Ariel reported five weeks later. "I drank the water, gave up coffee and diet soda and drank green tea instead, and made sure to include plenty of salad with fresh herbs, olive oil, and brightly colored fruits and vegetables. Not only did I not gain weight, I had all this energy and actually started going to the gym again. And I took the supplements, morning and evening."

Ariel's skin literally glowed. The anti-inflammatory foods, supplements, and rejuvenating powers of the polysaccharide peptide food helped repair and restore her complexion from the inside out. She had also lost the gaunt and haggard look that she was beginning to develop. Much to my delight, the skin around her mouth and chin now had a smoother, more toned, and firmer appearance.

"I could hardly believe it, but I saw immediate results in my skin from the first application of the topical peptides," Ariel continued. "That's what motivated me to follow the entire program—in fact, I thought I was going to have an accident on the LA freeway because I could not stop admiring my new face in the rearview mirror!"

What Lies Beneath:
It All Comes Back to Inflammation

Neuropeptides are powerful messengers that deliver their message to all cells in your body. Because of their amazing and beneficial properties, you can set them to the task of naturally, safely, and rapidly helping the skin to achieve optimum health and beauty.

Your skin is your body's first line of defense against a variety of environmental stressors, including those that are weather-related (such as temperature, humidity or lack of it, wind, heat, cold, and sunlight), as well as the many bacteria and chemicals that are abundant in today's world.

When it comes to chemicals, consider these facts. There are more than seventy-five thousand toxic chemicals classified by the EPA as potentially or definitely hazardous to human health. And new chemicals are being tested in the United States at the rate of six thousand or more per week. Dioxin, one of the deadliest substances known, is sprayed on coffee fields in Costa Rica. Mercury, besides leaking from dental fillings, is also found in fish, cosmetics, soil, pesticides, film, paint, and plastics. Arsenic may be present in coffee, some types of rice, salt, and smog. Cadmium is contained in cigarette smoke, coffee, gasoline, steel cooking pans, and metal pipes. Carbon monoxide gas, of course, comes from auto exhaust, cigarette smoke, and smog. Lead is found in dyes, gasoline, paint, plumbing, pottery, insecticides, tobacco smoke, textiles, and scrap metal. Many of these chemicals are also in our water, our food, and the air we breathe! The vast increase in chemicals in our environment, foods, and medicines has greatly altered our bodies' ability to rid themselves of toxins.

And the greater the number of toxins that are retained by the body, the greater the chances that they will cause inflammation, whether deep inside or on the surface of the skin.

Throughout these chapters and throughout my earlier books, *The Wrinkle Cure* and *The Perricone Prescription,* I repeatedly discussed the Inflammation–Aging–Disease Connection. That is, inflammation is at the basis of aging and at the basis of diverse degenerative diseases such as Alzheimer's, heart disease, cancer, arthritis, and autoimmune diseases. The same factors that cause these diverse diseases also affect the skin in outbreaks of problems such as acne, eczema, and shingles—and they're what give us wrinkles as well.

This can best be illustrated by examining the consequences of a lunchtime walk on a sunny summer day.

As the clock strikes noon, we turn away from our cluttered desk and computer screen, take a deep breath, and vow to forget the stressful workload for the next hour. We step out into the noonday sun, take a deep breath of the warm summer air, and derive great pleasure from the July afternoon.

While we bask in the almost tropical warmth, the sun is busy producing a full spectrum of electromagnetic radiation, ranging from the invisible, such as ultraviolet and infrared, to the visible portions of sunlight. Our skin begins soaking up the rays by absorbing this radiation, immediately placing the skin cells under stress. This happens because when sunlight strikes the skin, it results in the production of free radicals, which are missing one of their electrons in their outer orbit. Electrons, like people, like to travel in pairs. And so the free radical wants to complete its pair, and it does this by stealing an electron from one of the molecules in our skin cells. This results in a domino effect in which one free radical produces another, and another, and so on. This activity has harmful consequences for our cells because it increases pro-inflammatory chemicals—which generate even more free radicals.

Luckily, our cells do have a defense system made up of antioxidants (such as vitamins C and E and CoQ10), which will give up an electron to the free radical, completing its pair and thus preventing destruction to our skin cells. However, antioxidants are rapidly used up when we are exposed to the sun. The bad news is that with just one hour of exposure during our noontime walk, approximately 80 percent of the vitamin C stores in our skin are depleted.

In addition, these vitamins cannot provide complete protection from the inflammatory consequences of the sunlight. The outer portion of the cell, known as the cell plasma membrane, is readily attacked by these sunlight-induced free radicals. This results in the release of a fatty acid called arachidonic acid, which is quickly turned into powerful inflammation-causing chemicals.

These free radicals also stimulate the production of a compound in our cells called nuclear factor kappa B (NFkB), which in turn switches on the production of damaging compounds, influencing microscarring. As we continue our walk in the sun, another messenger in the cell, AP-1, is also activated by sunlight. AP-1 signals the cell to produce enzymes, which break down collagen, which then results in more microscarring and—you guessed it—more visible wrinkles. What you need to understand is that free radicals themselves do very little damage to the skin. Instead, they trigger an inflammatory response and kick off a chain of chemical events that can go on for hours, weeks, or months. The result? Damage to important portions of the cell, such as the mitochondria, which are responsible for energy production. This causes the cell to break down without the energy it needs to repair itself.

And if you think you have to be sunbathing on the beach to trigger these harmful effects, you're (sadly) mistaken. This entire process, starting with the walk out into the noonday sun and ending with the activation of collagen-digesting enzymes, takes about five minutes. Once again, inflammation is the final common pathway to this dermal wound that becomes a visible wrinkle. Understanding this process allows us to formulate various therapeutic interventions that will minimize or prevent inflammation and subsequent wrinkling of the skin.

Alpha Lipoic Acid to the Rescue

Alpha lipoic acid (ALA), which occurs naturally inside the body's mitochondria, is called the universal antioxidant because it is both fat and water soluble. That means it is easily absorbed through the layers of the skin and works equally well as a free-radical fighter in both the cell plasma membrane and the watery interior of the cell. To illustrate its effectiveness as an antioxidant: It is four hundred times stronger than vitamins E and C combined. ALA also boosts energy production by helping the mitochondria convert food to energy. Whether you take ALA as a supplement or apply it topically in a lotion, it performs as an antioxidant while it increases cellular metabolism.

The good news is that alpha lipoic acid inhibits the activation of NFkB better than any other antioxidant. It blocks the production of enzymes that damage the collagen fibers, preserving a smooth skin surface. It is equally effective in preventing glycation, the harmful effects of sugar molecules on collagen fibers.

ALA also has a tremendous effect on the transcription factor AP-1. As mentioned, when AP-1 is turned on by the oxidative stress created by our walk in the sunlight, it turns on production of enzymes that actually digest collagen, causing microscars—resulting in the birth of a wrinkle.

However, when AP-1 is activated by alpha lipoic acid, it signals the AP-1 to digest *damaged* collagen, resulting in the elimination and erasure of wrinkles.

Alpha lipoic acid's powerful anti-glycation, anti-wrinkle properties are discussed in chapter 7, the supplement chapter. There are no good food sources of ALA, so the best ways to maximize its benefits are to take it as a supplement and to use it topically in skin care products. I recommend applying an ALA topical product daily, in the morning under your moisturizer and makeup.

WHERE TO FIND PRODUCTS WITH ALPHA LIPOIC ACID

There are many skin care products available now that contain alpha lipoic acid. Here is a short list of retail and Internet sites that offer these products:

- N. V. Perricone, M.D., Ltd., Flagship Store at 791 Madison Avenue (at 67th Street), New York, NY; www.nvperriconemd.com
- Nordstrom; www.nordstrom.com
- Sephora; www.sephora.com
- Selected Neiman Marcus; www.neimanmarcus.com
- Selected Saks; www.saksfifthavenue.com
- Henri Bendel
- Clyde's on Madison

A Revolution in Skin Rejuvenation: Topical Peptide Products

Perhaps the greatest breakthrough in skin care and rejuvenation to come along in years is the development of topical peptide products.

These products came out of the discovery that peptides and neuropeptides produced by the thymus gland stimulate the production of collagen and elastin, both of which are helpful in healing wounds. If we look upon wrinkles as microscopic wounds, logic then dictates that thymic peptides would be beneficial in "healing" wrinkles and other signs of aging skin.

THE FRACTION FIVE

Although there have been dozens of biologically active peptides isolated from the thymus gland, early studies were carried out with an extract of thymus known as *Fraction Five*. Fraction Five contains more than forty different peptides, many of which have powerful biologic activity.

One important peptide found in Fraction Five is called *thymosin beta 4*. What makes this molecule so important for youthful and beautiful skin is its function in healing wounds. As we age, it is more difficult for wounds to heal. Wound healing is also a problem for diabetics and bedridden patients. In order for a wound to heal, the body goes through several steps. Ironically, the critical initial step in wound healing is inflammation. Inflammation results in increased blood flow to the wound and production of various growth factors, which will promote closure of the wound. So initially we see inflammation, followed by increased blood flow (or restriction of blood flow if bleeding is profuse), followed by angiogenesis (the growth of new blood vessels), followed by the migration of skin cells known as fibroblasts to the area. The fibroblasts lay down new collagen, which helps remodel the damaged tissue.

Thymosin beta 4 plays a role in many of these steps, such as increased blood vessel growth, modulation of the inflammatory response, and migration of the skin cells into the wound, as well as stimulating production of collagen and elastin. Thymosin beta 4 can also act as a powerful anti-inflammatory agent, protecting vulnerable tissue from the effects of inflammation that is out of control.

The Miracle of Neuropeptides and the Skin

In studies applying various neuropeptide preparations directly to the skin, exciting clinical benefits were observed almost immediately upon application. Within minutes of applying a topical cream containing multiple neuropeptides and DMAE, a powerful anti-inflammatory with activity in both skin and brain, we see:

- A visible increase in radiance and glow to the skin. This is the result of the compounds' powerful anti–inflammatory activity, as well as their effects on blood circulation and cell metabolism.
- An increase in firmness, because the neuropeptides aid in collagen and elastin production.
- Improved appearance of the skin's resilience, tone, and texture.
- Decreased appearance of fine lines and wrinkles.
- Decreased appearance of tiny veins and capillaries.
- Maximized regeneration and hydration of the skin.

As we get older, our skin cell turnover decreases, we lose the thickness of the dermis through the loss of collagen and elastin, and we experience a decrease in important blood vessels that carry nutrients to the skin cells—all of which can be greatly ameliorated by the application of topical peptides.

I recommend daily application to the face and neck. Topical peptides can be applied along with a moisturizer and/or sunscreen.

The results of the application of topical neuropeptides are the most impressive I have seen in my twenty years of research. The neuropeptide topical formulas I have developed contain multiple peptides delivered in a special base that allows the molecules to penetrate the skin, where they can activate receptor sites and achieve maximum benefits.

WHERE TO FIND
TOPICAL NEUROPEPTIDES

There are many peptide products on the market; however, I cannot vouch for most of them, because I have not tested them. Here is a short list of retailers and Internet sites that offer neuropeptide products. Read labels carefully: If the stated content is "pentapeptides," this is vastly different from "neuropeptides," which have to be synthesized on an individual basis. Baked Barley at the following:

- **N. V. Perricone, M.D., Ltd., Flagship Store at 791 Madison Avenue (at 67th Street), New York, NY; www.nvperriconemd.com**
- **Nordstrom; www.nordstrom.com**
- **Sephora; www.sephora.com**
- **Selected Neiman Marcus; www.neimanmarcus.com**
- **Selected Saks; www.saksfifthavenue.com**
- **Henri Bendel**
- **Clyde's on Madison**

The science of peptides and neuropeptides, while not new, is still in its infancy. It is a field of science that is attracting the brightest and best minds. Every day, research unlocks new findings on the roles peptides and neuropeptides play and how we can best put them to work for us. As part of the 28-Day Program you will find in the next chapter, I provide you with a simple three-tiered program of anti-inflammatory food, supplements, and topical treatments as a way to incorporate their superior attributes and benefits into your daily life.

PART III

THE 28-DAY PERRICONE PROGRAM

Now you know all the key elements that go into this program: rainbow foods, superfoods, herbs and spices, polysaccharides, and supplements. Every one of these elements is essential. Add in exercise, which I'll discuss in the next chapter, and you've got the makings of a new, healthy way to live your life. And you will understand the science behind the program and why each of the elements is so important to its success.

If you find it too difficult to make all these changes at once, don't. Start by slowly subtracting some bad habits (drinking coffee, smoking cigarettes, not getting enough sleep) and adding in some good ones (including more fish in your diet, taking one or two of the recommended supplements, using a topical neuropeptide cream). Try some of the recipes in appendix A. They're very healthy, and they're delicious, too. As soon as you begin to make these small changes, you'll find the program easier and easier to follow. Your energy will increase dramatically during the day. You'll sleep better at night. Within just a few days, you will look and feel so much better that your goal will be to make the 28-Day Program a way of life for you.

The 28-Day Perricone Program

Nothing great was ever achieved without enthusiasm.
— RALPH WALDO EMERSON

ONE OF THE JOYS OF INTRODUCING my patients and readers to the Perricone Promise is witnessing the enthusiasm they develop right from the start. Because dramatic results can be seen so quickly—in as little as three days—they are inspired to stay with the program and integrate it into their lives.

Every day, I learn something new about the powerful interaction between the foods we eat and the rate at which we age. In this chapter, I have outlined a simple, balanced menu and supplement plan that will provide the following benefits:

- Prevent swings in blood sugar levels.
- Increase the beauty and health of your skin and internal organs.
- Increase memory and brain power.
- Keep your emotional well-being at optimum levels.
- Energize the whole person.
- Optimize the function of your immune system.

I led the list with the all-important mantra of keeping blood sugar levels balanced because if you eat or drink foods that cause a rapid rise in blood sugar, you set off a cascade of chemical reactions that create inflammation. By learning how to suppress the pro-inflamma-

173

tory peptides, while stimulating the anti-inflammatory peptides through diet and supplements, you have a critically important new tool for achieving this goal.

This is a program that is meant to keep you healthy for life. Once the twenty-eight days are gone, you can't just return to your old wicked ways. The thing is, you won't want to. Your skin will look better than it has in years. You will have energy and a youthful vitality. And you will probably lose excess fat as you go.

In fact, one of the often unexpected yet welcome benefits of following the dietary guidelines in *The Perricone Promise* is a loss of excess weight. Many men and women discover (often for the first time) that they lose weight and gain energy without self-denial, hunger, or feelings of deprivation.

What's the secret? Keeping your blood sugar levels even while keeping your metabolism stimulated. Sudden upward spikes in blood sugar levels—caused by eating sweet or starchy foods such as pasta, potatoes, pastries, candy, soda, and juice—actually prevent you from burning fat because they place a "lock" on your cells' fat-burning mechanism. In addition, the empty calories in these types of foods leave you craving more as soon as your blood sugar level drops—which it is guaranteed to do. When you eat low-glycemic carbohydrates and quality fats and protein, you don't have blood sugar swings, so overeating and food cravings are greatly reduced. Also, when you go for long periods without eating, your metabolism all but shuts down to conserve fat stores and energy. Thus, skipping meals can have the opposite effect of what you intend if you are looking to take off a few (or more than a few) pounds.

Achieving and maintaining a healthy weight is not just about beauty. Excess fat has a direct impact on the Beauty–Brain Connection. The thymus gland, for instance, influences the production of stress hormones. Too many stress hormones and you'll try to calm yourself with foods that give you short-term mood and energy boosts: sugars and starches. After the initial rise in serotonin (the "feel-good" hormone), levels drop, resulting in a vicious cycle of craving pro-inflammatory, fattening, and wrinkle-inducing foods. The foods and supplements on the 28-Day Program also help decrease the harmful effects of stress hormones, such as cortisol, which cause you to store body fat, particularly in the abdominal area. In addition, these anti-inflammatory food choices reduce the cravings for junk foods that keep you in dangerous insulin spike-and-drop cycles. If you are overweight, you increase your risk of many diseases, including diabetes, high blood pressure, heart disease, and stroke. We now know that each fat cell produces inflammatory chemicals that then circulate throughout the body, increasing the risk of aging and age-related diseases.

Another factor in weight control is consuming foods that are rich in fiber. Fiber has a great many benefits, not the least of which is its ability to slow absorption of foods, helping to keep those all-important blood sugar levels on an even keel. This was given serious consideration in the 28-Day Program, which is why it contains many recipes utilizing foods rich in both soluble and insoluble fiber— including barley, oats, lentils and beans, and liberal amounts of fresh fruit and vegetables.

Exercise for Health

Exercise is also an important factor in regulating neuropeptides. In the 1980s, the neuropeptide beta-endorphin was found to be a significant pain reducer and appeared to promote feelings of euphoria and exhilaration while reducing feelings of depression and anxiety. This phenomenon has since become known as the runner's high, because beta-endorphin is synthesized during aerobic types of activity, particularly running. This may be one of the key reasons that exercise is such an important stress reducer: It appears to stimulate the production of the neuropeptides that contribute to feelings of happiness, as opposed to the neuropeptide Substance P (for example), which causes feelings of depression and anxiety.

But aerobics aren't the only kinds of exercise with health benefits. The Perricone Promise Program recommends blending three distinct types of exercise:

1. Weight resistance
2. Cardiovascular/aerobic
3. Flexibility

For optimum benefits, incorporate all three into your regimen. You can rotate among the three to keep your routine interesting and challenging.

1. Weight training and/or weight lifting is an excellent way to build muscle and strength. Weight training builds strength by way of progressive resistance training: The resistance, or weight, is increased as the muscles develop. Believe it or not, this is also part of the Brain–Beauty Connection. Resistance training releases growth hormone while it lowers stress and its accompanying level of cortisol. Before starting a weight training program (if you are new to this form of exercise), consult your physician and/or a professional trainer to avoid injury and to ensure that you are performing the exercises correctly.

2. Cardiovascular/aerobic exercises such as running, jogging, in-line skating, kickboxing, biking, hiking, and swimming greatly increase endurance and stamina as well as energy and well-being. Aerobics are weight training for the heart—a muscle that pumps blood throughout the body. This muscle is strengthened by aerobic exercise, which allows the heart to deliver more oxygen to the body. The latest research shows that you don't have to be an extreme athlete to get aerobic benefits; all you need are three aerobic exercise sessions a week, of twenty to thirty minutes each. Once again, do not start any exercise program that increases your heart rate unless you have consulted your physician or are already following an exercise regimen.

3. Finally, exercises that increase flexibility should be incorporated into your regimen. A number of disciplines actually have both cardiovascular/aerobic and flexibility benefits, including the martial arts, kickboxing, dancing, gymnastics, and swimming.

PILATES

Pilates is an outstanding way to increase strength and flexibility without building bulk. This has made the Pilates Method very popılar with dancers—in fact, some of the first people to use the Pilates Method were two famous pioneers in the world of dance, Martha Graham and George Balanchine.

Pilates was developed in the 1920s by the legendary physical trainer and founder of the Pilates Studio Joseph H. Pilates. It is a series of controlled movements engaging your body and mind, performed on specifically designed exercise apparatus and supervised by extensively trained teachers. To learn more, go to www.pilates-studio.com.

According to the excellent and informative Web site, the Pilates Method:

- Provides a method of body conditioning that promotes physical harmony and balance.
- Is effective for people of all ages and physical conditions.
- Provides a refreshing and energizing workout.
- Can be personalized, in one-on-one conditioning sessions.
- Is appropriate regardless of current fitness level.
- Can be integrated into rehabilitative exercise and physical therapy programs.
- Is safe for pregnant women, because it will teach them proper breathing and body alignment, as well as helping improve concentration and recover body shape and tone after pregnancy.

Important Tips for the Perricone Promise 28-Day Program

- Eat your protein first at each meal and snack. The best protein sources are cold-water fish such as salmon and halibut.
- Use fresh and dried herbs and spices liberally—oregano, ginger, cayenne pepper, basil, marjoram, turmeric, garlic, cinnamon. All these foods perform many age-fighting functions ranging from antioxidant, anti-inflammatory activities to regulation of blood sugar.
- For *new* anti-aging breakthroughs, think *ancient* cuisine. Authentic foods from the Mediterranean, India, and the Near,

Middle, and Far East provide amazing anti-aging benefits. These include simple curries loaded with turmeric, a vast array of lentil dishes, and enough aromatic herbs and spices to turn every meal into an antioxidant powerhouse. Avoid dishes calling for cream or ghee—stick with the more simple, healthful ingredients. Always include a quality source of protein at every meal and snack.

- Don't forget the fiber. Make sure that all your carbohydrate choices are high in fiber. Studies have shown that dietary fiber —including foods such as apples, barley, beans, lentils and other legumes, fruits and vegetables, old-fashioned oatmeal, and oat bran—lowers blood cholesterol. Because they are more slowly digested, these foods will *not* cause a rise in blood sugar. A diet rich in high-fiber foods is indispensable in controlling unwanted weight gain.

- Drink eight to ten glasses of water every day. Constipation can result as you increase fiber intake if your water intake is not adequate.

- Choose organic, free-range chicken and turkey for superior flavor and to avoid the antibiotics and processing of regular commercially raised poultry.

- Choose eggs from cage-free chickens that are fed diets high in the omega-3s, such as flaxseed. These eggs are now widely available and are a much healthier choice than conventional eggs.

- Buy organic. Pesticides can leave toxic residues on plants that can harm your organ systems.

- Choose wild Alaskan salmon over farm-raised.

- In addition to eating liberal amounts of wild Alaskan salmon, introduce anchovies and sardines into your diet—these tiny fish deliver enormous health and beauty benefits. They are rich sources of the omega-3 essential fatty acids, and because they are low on the food chain, they are less contaminated than larger fish. They also contain DMAE to help keep skin toned and firm. A great way to introduce anchovies is to add anchovy paste (or mash a few anchovies) to your salad dressing. This is particularly delicious and an important staple of the original Caesar salad—just remember to hold the croutons!

- Sauté foods over medium heat and *do not brown* the food. The browning reaction is the result of glycation, in which the proteins cross-link. A study published in the *Proceedings of the National Academy of Sciences* revealed that eating foods cooked at high temperature may increase the rate at which we age. According to this study, the ingestion of high-temperature-cooked foods causes chronic inflammation and the formation of advanced glycation end-products (also appropriately named AGEs). For more on this, refer to chapter 7.

- I recommend having a yogurt or kefir smoothie with açaí and berries (blueberries, blackberries, raspberries, or strawberries), or a tablespoon of POM Wonderful pomegranate extract, *once a day*—for breakfast or as one of your snacks. This is an outstanding way to add protein, calcium, potassium, phosphorus, vitamins B_6 and B_{12}, niacin, folic acid, and potassium to your diet, in addition to the all-important probiotic (health-promoting, anti-aging intestinal flora) antioxidant properties of the açaí and the berries.

- Liberally garnish your savory dishes with chopped scallions, chopped chives, and other members of the onion family, for both their unique flavors and their outstanding health benefits.

- Don't forget the sprouts. Broccoli sprouts are exceptionally high in antioxidants. All sprouts, however, from alfalfa to sunflower, and lentil to radish, offer outstanding health benefits and add flavor to salads, stir-fries, wraps, even soups and stews. Sprouts are widely available in natural food markets and finer supermarkets.

- When choosing lettuce for salads, the darker green, the better. Choose romaine, mixed baby greens, mesclun, arugula, kale, spinach, escarole, broccoli rabe, or the like. Avoid iceberg.

- Add leftover cooked veggies to salads. Cooked broccoli, for example, tastes great when dressed with extra-virgin olive oil and fresh lemon juice.

- Nuts and seeds also make a great addition to salads and stir-fries.
- If you want radiant, supple skin, don't go low-fat or fat-free! After water, fat is the most abundant substance in your body. Fats from animal and vegetable sources provide a concentrated source of energy in the diet; they also provide the building blocks for cell membranes, for hormones, and for prostaglandins. In addition, they act as carriers for important fat-soluble vitamins A, D, E, and K. Dietary fats are needed for the conversion of carotene to vitamin A and for a host of other processes. More than 70 percent of your brain and nerve cells are made of fat, making this critical tissue resilient and shock-resistant. Every cell membrane in your body is at least 30 percent fat. Both cholesterol and saturated fat are essential for growth in babies and children. In babies, fat is needed in the formation of myelin—a specialized membrane that protects the nerves and is essential to the normal development of the central nervous system and the brain. The fat contained in breast milk best meets this development need. Healthy fats include those found in fish such as salmon, in nuts and seeds, yogurt and kefir, and olive oil.
- Cottage cheese is an excellent food, but supermarket brands contain ingredients that are undesirable, ranging from preservatives such as potassium sorbate to guar gum, carrageenan, fillers, and stabilizers. Try to purchase at natural food markets where there are no ingredients other than cultured pasteurized Grade A milk, cream, and salt. Also look for brands that are made from the milk of cows that have not been given hormones or antibiotics.

The 28-Day Perricone Program

Before you begin the program, there are a few things you should know. Of course, before making any dietary or physical changes to your daily regimen, you should consult your physician. Now, here are the basics of the Perricone Promise: It's important to begin your day with a peptide boost—that's why I recommend taking a polysaccharide peptide food such as peptide functional food powder (PEP) or a maitake mushroom supplement first thing in the morning. Then, directly after your shower, apply a neuropeptide cream (see chapter 8) to your face and throat. That should start you off looking great and keep you looking young and radiant all day.

Now that you're eating healthier, you'll be getting more vitamins and nutrients into your system every day. However, I advise a basic supplement regimen to help improve your chances of balancing your hormones, boosting your peptides, and enhancing the results obtained by combining all parts of the 28-Day Program. Regardless of which products you choose, remember to look for a comprehensive formula that contains vitamins A, C, and E, alpha lipoic acid, the essential fatty acids, and the complete spectrum of B vitamins and minerals including calcium and magnesium (see the Resource Guide for reputable manufacturers).

You can take each of these supplements separately, or you can take them in multivitamin combinations. When buying supplements, read labels carefully to find out just what ingredients are included, as well as their dosages. There is another option, and that is to take ready-made packets of supplements, such as the Total Skin and Body Packet that I have developed, which includes what I feel is the optimum combination of supplements for an anti-inflammation, anti-aging program.

Neuropeptide Supplement Tablet Dosage: Take one neuropeptide supplement tablet with breakfast and one with lunch for twelve days. After that, cut the dosage to one neuropeptide supplement tablet per day, or every other day.

Maitake Uses and Dosage: Both the D-Fraction and the SX-Fraction are available in either capsule form or as an extract. Follow the directions on the label or from your health care provider. Maitake D-Fraction contains a unique polysaccharide compound that supports immune cell function. The dosage is two capsules twice a day between meals. Maitake D-Fraction is specially geared for people who seek enhanced immune system function.

Maitake SX-Fraction is the first dietary supplement of its class that specifically addresses its beneficial role in Syndrome X as a part of a diet to help maintain healthy blood sugar and blood pressure levels. If you're more interested in protecting your immune system, choose Maitake D-Fraction; if you're concerned about Syndrome X, choose Maitake SX-Fraction.

WEEK ONE

Remember, every meal and snack should have three important nutrients:

- Protein
- Low-glycemic carbohydrates
- Essential fats

The larger amounts of protein are for those who are physically active or larger and therefore have more muscle mass. In any meal or snack, you can substitute a can of wild Alaskan salmon for the suggested protein source for the sake of convenience. See the Resource Guide for salmon sources.

DAY 1. Monday

Start the day with 1 teaspoon peptide functional food powder mixed with 6 ounces water or Maitake Fraction-D or Fraction-SX.
Exercise for the day.
After cleansing, apply neuropeptide cream to face and throat.

Breakfast
1 soft-boiled egg
½ cup cottage cheese topped with 1 tablespoon ground flaxseed
⅛–¼ cup (measure before cooking) old-fashioned oatmeal with
   ½ teaspoon cinnamon
¼ cup berries
8 ounces green tea or water

Supplements: Daily supplement regimen, 2 high-quality Norwegian fish oil capsules, 1 neuropeptide supplement

Lunch

¾ cup Ginger Chicken or Tofu Salad (see the recipe in appendix A)
1 kiwi fruit
8 ounces water

Supplements: Daily supplement regimen, 2 high-quality Norwegian fish oil capsules, 1 neuropeptide supplement

Snack

6 ounces plain yogurt or kefir mixed with 1 serving açaí
3 almonds
8 ounces water

Dinner

Hazelnut-Encrusted Wild Salmon Fillets on a Bed of Wilted
Greens (see the recipe in appendix A)
2-inch wedge cantaloupe
8 ounces water
2 high-quality Norwegian fish oil capsules

Bedtime

1 hard-boiled egg
1 apple
3 walnuts
8 ounces water

DAY 2. Tuesday

Start the day with 1 teaspoon peptide functional food powder mixed with 6 ounces water or Maitake Fraction-D or Fraction-SX. After cleansing, apply neuropeptide cream to face and throat.

Breakfast
Omelet made with 2 whole eggs, 2 egg whites, and fresh herbs
Yogurt or kefir smoothie—6 ounces plain yogurt, 1 tablespoon
ground flaxseed, ¼ cup mixed berries, and 1 serving açaí
8 ounces green tea or water

Supplements: Daily supplement regimen, 2 high-quality Norwegian fish oil capsules, 1 neuropeptide supplement

Lunch
Greek Salad Topped with Grilled Chicken, Salmon, Shrimp, or
Tofu (see the recipe in appendix A)
1 apple
8 ounces water

Supplements: Daily supplement regimen, 2 high-quality Norwegian fish oil capsules, 1 neuropeptide supplement

Snack
½ cup cottage cheese topped with 1 tablespoon ground flaxseed
1 pear
8 ounces water

Dinner
1 bowl Rich Lentil and Turkey Sausage Soup (see the recipe in
appendix A)
1 cup dark green leafy salad with 3–6 ounces grilled chicken
dressed with olive oil and lemon juice to taste and ½ cup
sprouts
8 ounces water
2 high-quality Norwegian fish oil capsules

Bedtime
1–2 ounces sliced roast turkey or chicken breast
1 tablespoon raw pumpkin seeds
2-inch wedge honeydew melon
8 ounces water

DAY 3. Wednesday

Start the day with 1 teaspoon peptide functional food powder mixed with 6 ounces water or Maitake Fraction-D or Fraction-SX.
Exercise for the day.
After cleansing, apply neuropeptide cream to face and throat.

Breakfast
 4–8 ounces grilled or smoked salmon
 ½ cup cooked barley with ½ teaspoon cinnamon topped with 1
   tablespoon berries
 8 ounces green tea or water

Supplements: Daily supplement regimen, 2 high-quality Norwegian fish oil capsules, 1 neuropeptide supplement

Lunch
 Jumbo Shrimp Cocktail (see the recipe in appendix A)
 ½ avocado
 1 apple
 8 ounces water

Supplements: Daily supplement regimen, 2 high-quality Norwegian fish oil capsules, 1 neuropeptide supplement

Snack
 6 ounces plain yogurt mixed with 1 serving açaí
 1 tablespoon sunflower seeds
 8 ounces water

Dinner
 Chicken Almond Ding (see the recipe in appendix A)
 ½ cup fruit salad with mixed berries, kiwi, and pear
 8 ounces water
 2 high-quality Norwegian fish oil capsules

Bedtime

¼ cup Hummus (see the recipe in appendix A)
1 celery stalk
8 ounces water

DAY 4. Thursday

Start the day with 1 teaspoon peptide functional food powder mixed with 6 ounces water or Maitake Fraction-D or Fraction-SX. Exercise for the day.
After cleansing, apply neuropeptide cream to face and throat.

Breakfast

Feta cheese omelet—2 whole eggs, 2 egg whites, ½ ounce crumbled feta, and ¼ teaspoon dry or fresh dill weed
2-inch wedge cantaloupe
8 ounces green tea or water

Supplements: Daily supplement regimen, 2 high-quality Norwegian fish oil capsules, 1 neuropeptide supplement

Lunch

Crab or Lobster Cocktail (see the recipe in appendix A)
Green salad dressed with extra-virgin olive oil and lemon juice to taste
1 pear
8 ounces water

Supplements: Daily supplement regimen, 2 high-quality Norwegian fish oil capsules, 1 neuropeptide supplement

Snack

Kefir smoothie—mix in blender 6 ounces unsweetened kefir, ¼ cup mixed berries, 1 teaspoon ground flaxseed, and 1 serving açaí
8 ounces water

Dinner

Curried Chicken or Tofu (see the recipe in appendix A) served
on ½ cup cooked barley
Cool and Creamy Cucumber Salad (see the recipe in appendix A)
8 ounces water
2 high-quality Norwegian fish oil capsules

Bedtime

1–2 ounces sliced turkey or chicken breast
¼ cup cherries
3 almonds
8 ounces water

DAY 5. Friday

Start the day with 1 teaspoon peptide functional food powder
mixed with 6 ounces water or Maitake Fraction-D or Fraction-SX.
Exercise for the day.
After cleansing, apply neuropeptide cream to face and throat.

Breakfast

1 soft-boiled egg
2 slices turkey bacon
Yogurt or kefir—mix in blender 6 ounces plain yogurt or kefir,
¼ cup mixed berries, and 1 serving açaí
8 ounces green tea or water

Supplements: Daily supplement regimen, 2 high-quality Norwegian fish oil capsules, 1 neuropeptide supplement

Lunch

Chicken, Turkey, or Tofu Salad Wrap (see the recipe in appendix A)
8 ounces water

Supplements: Daily supplement regimen, 2 high-quality Norwegian fish oil capsules, 1 neuropeptide supplement

Snack
  1 hard-boiled egg
  3 cherry tomatoes
  3 olives
  8 ounces water

Dinner
  Salmon Teriyaki (can also be made with chicken breast or tofu—
    see the recipe in appendix A)
  ½ cup steamed asparagus
  ½ cup lentils
  8 ounces water
  2 high-quality Norwegian fish oil capsules

Bedtime
  ½ cup cottage cheese
  1 tablespoon chopped pumpkin seeds
  8 ounces water

DAY 6. Saturday

Start the day with 1 teaspoon peptide functional food powder
mixed with 6 ounces water or Maitake Fraction-D or Fraction-SX.
  Exercise for the day.
  After cleansing, apply neuropeptide cream to face and throat.

Breakfast
  2 slices Canadian or turkey bacon
  ½ cup cottage cheese
  ½ cup Buckwheat Cereal (see the recipe in appendix A)
  1 kiwi
  8 ounces green tea or water

Supplements: Daily supplement regimen, 2 high-quality Norwegian fish oil capsules, 1 neuropeptide supplement

Lunch
½ cup Hummus (see the recipe in appendix A)
4–6 ounces broiled chicken, salmon, or tofu
2 celery stalks
1 apple

Supplements: Daily supplement regimen, 2 high-quality Norwegian fish oil capsules, 1 neuropeptide supplement

Snack
Yogurt—mix in blender 6 ounces plain yogurt and 1 serving açaí
3 walnuts
8 ounces water

Dinner
Grilled Indian Chicken (see the recipe in appendix A)
½ cup Baked Barley (see the recipe in appendix A)
2-inch wedge cantaloupe
8 ounces water
2 high-quality Norwegian fish oil capsules

Bedtime
1–2 ounces sliced turkey or chicken breast
¼ cup pumpkin seeds
½ cup cherries
8 ounces water

DAY 7. Sunday

Start the day with 1 teaspoon peptide functional food powder mixed with 6 ounces water or Maitake Fraction-D or Fraction-SX.
Exercise for the day: Relaxation.
After cleansing, apply neuropeptide cream to face and throat.

Breakfast
3–6 ounces broiled or smoked salmon
⅛–¼ cup (measure before cooking) old-fashioned oatmeal with
½ teaspoon cinnamon

1 kiwi fruit

8 ounces green tea or water

Supplements: Daily supplement regimen, 2 high-quality Norwegian fish oil capsules, 1 neuropeptide supplement

Lunch

Turkey Burger (see the recipe in appendix A)

Green salad dressed with extra-virgin olive oil and lemon juice to taste

½ cup berries

8 ounces water

Supplements: Daily supplement regimen, 2 high-quality Norwegian fish oil capsules, 1 neuropeptide supplement

Snack

½ cup cottage cheese topped with 1 tablespoon ground flaxseed

1 apple

8 ounces water

Dinner

Savory Halibut with Braised Red Peppers and Leeks (see the recipe in appendix A)

½ cup Buckwheat Pilaf (see the recipe in appendix A)

8 ounces water

2 high-quality Norwegian fish oil capsules

Bedtime

1–2 ounces sliced turkey or chicken breast

3 olives

3 strawberries

8 ounces water

WEEK TWO

DAY 8. Monday

Start the day with 1 teaspoon peptide functional food powder mixed with 6 ounces water or Maitake Fraction-D or Fraction-SX.
Exercise for the day.
After cleansing, apply neuropeptide cream to face and throat.

Breakfast
Omelet made with 2 whole eggs, 2 egg whites, fresh herbs, and chopped chives or scallions
Yogurt or kefir smoothie—mix in blender 6 ounces unsweetened kefir, ¼ cup mixed berries, 1 teaspoon ground flaxseed, and 1 serving açaí
8 ounces green tea or water

Supplements: Daily supplement regimen, 2 high-quality Norwegian fish oil capsules, 1 neuropeptide supplement

Lunch
Jumbo Shrimp, Crab, or Lobster Cocktail (see the recipe in appendix A)
Green salad dressed with extra-virgin olive oil and lemon juice to taste, garnished with ½ avocado
1 pear
8 ounces water

Supplements: Daily supplement regimen, 2 high-quality Norwegian fish oil capsules, 1 neuropeptide supplement

Snack
½ cup cottage cheese topped with 1 tablespoon chopped sunflower or pumpkin seeds
1 apple
8 ounces water

Dinner

Lemon Chicken (see the recipe in appendix A)

Saffron-Scented Oat Pilaf with Parsley (see the recipe in
appendix A)

Mixed fruit plate with thinly sliced melon, kiwi, apple

8 ounces water

2 high-quality Norwegian fish oil capsules

Bedtime

1–2 ounces sliced turkey or chicken breast

3 almonds

¼ cup blueberries

8 ounces water

DAY 9. Tuesday

Start the day with 1 teaspoon peptide functional food powder
mixed with 6 ounces water or Maitake Fraction-D or Fraction-SX.

Exercise for the day.

After cleansing, apply neuropeptide cream to face and throat.

Breakfast

Omelet made with 2 whole eggs and 2 egg whites filled with
½ cup sautéed onions and mushrooms

2-inch wedge honeydew melon

8 ounces green tea or water

Supplements: Daily supplement regimen, 2 high-quality Norwegian fish oil capsules, 1 neuropeptide supplement

Lunch

Hearty Chicken Soup (see the recipe in appendix A)

1 pear

8 ounces water

Supplements: Daily supplement regimen, 2 high-quality Norwegian fish oil capsules, 1 neuropeptide supplement

Snack
1–2 ounces turkey breast
3 walnuts
1 apple
8 ounces water

Dinner
Baked Scrod with Tomato-Basil Sauce (see the recipe in appendix A)
Spinach with Garlic and Ginger (see the recipe in appendix A)
½ cup Baked Barley (see the recipe in appendix A)
¼ cup berries
8 ounces water
2 high-quality Norwegian fish oil capsules

Bedtime
½ cup cottage cheese topped with 1 tablespoon ground flaxseed
¼ cup cherries
8 ounces water

DAY 10. Wednesday

Start the day with 1 teaspoon peptide functional food powder mixed with 6 ounces water or Maitake Fraction-D or Fraction-SX.
Exercise for the day.
After cleansing, apply neuropeptide cream to face and throat.

Breakfast
3–6 ounces grilled or baked salmon fillet or lox
Yogurt or kefir smoothie—mix in blender 6 ounces unsweetened kefir, ¼ cup mixed berries, and 1 serving açaí

3 macadamia nuts
8 ounces green tea or water

Supplements: Daily supplement regimen, 2 high-quality Norwegian fish oil capsules, 1 neuropeptide supplement

Lunch
Chicken, Turkey, or Tofu Salad Wrap (see the recipe in appendix A)
Large green salad with sliced tomatoes
2-inch wedge cantaloupe
8 ounces water

Supplements: Daily supplement regimen, 2 high-quality Norwegian fish oil capsules, 1 neuropeptide supplement

Snack
½ cup Hummus (see the recipe in appendix A)
2 celery stalks
3 almonds
8 ounces water

Dinner
Curried Shrimp (see the recipe in appendix A)
½ cup cooked whole oats or barley—cooked in the same
    manner as brown rice
1 cup salad made with mixed baby greens and ½ avocado,
    dressed with extra-virgin olive oil and lemon juice to taste
8 ounces water
2 high-quality Norwegian fish oil capsules

Bedtime
1–2 ounces sliced chicken or turkey breast
¼ cup pumpkin seeds
1 apple
8 ounces water

DAY 11. Thursday

Start the day with 1 teaspoon peptide functional food powder mixed with 6 ounces water or Maitake Fraction-D or Fraction-SX.
Exercise for the day.
After cleansing, apply neuropeptide cream to face and throat.

Breakfast
Omelet made with 2 eggs and 2 egg whites, fresh herbs, and 1 ounce feta cheese
⅛–¼ cup (measure before cooking) old-fashioned oatmeal topped with 1 tablespoon chopped pumpkin seeds
1 kiwi fruit
8 ounces green tea or water

Supplements: Daily supplement regimen, 2 high-quality Norwegian fish oil capsules, 1 neuropeptide supplement

Lunch
Salmon Burger on a Bed of Baby Greens (see the recipe in appendix A)
1 apple
8 ounces water

Supplements: Daily supplement regimen, 2 high-quality Norwegian fish oil capsules, 1 neuropeptide supplement

Snack
Yogurt or kefir smoothie—mix in blender 6 ounces unsweetened kefir, ¼ cup mixed berries, 1 teaspoon ground flaxseed, and 1 serving açaí
8 ounces green tea or water

Dinner
Two-Bean Turkey or Tofu Chili (see the recipe in appendix A)
Green salad dressed with extra-virgin olive oil and lemon juice to taste

1 pear
8 ounces water
2 high-quality Norwegian fish oil capsules

Bedtime

½ cup cottage cheese topped with 1 teaspoon flaxseed
¼ cup berries
8 ounces water

DAY 12. Friday

Start the day with 1 teaspoon peptide functional food powder mixed with 6 ounces water or Maitake Fraction-D or Fraction-SX. Exercise for the day.

After cleansing, apply neuropeptide cream to face and throat.

Breakfast

2 links turkey or tofu sausage
2 soft-boiled eggs
½ cup cooked barley topped with 1 tablespoon yogurt and
   ¼ cup berries
8 ounces green tea or water

Supplements: Daily supplement regimen, 2 high-quality Norwegian fish oil capsules, 1 neuropeptide supplement

Lunch

Mediterranean Turkey Soup (see the recipe in appendix A)
3 walnuts
2-inch wedge cantaloupe

Supplements: Daily supplement regimen, 2 high-quality Norwegian fish oil capsules, 1 neuropeptide supplement

Snack

Yogurt or kefir smoothie—mix in blender 6 ounces unsweetened
kefir, ¼ cup mixed berries, 1 teaspoon ground flaxseed, and 1
serving açaí

8 ounces water

Dinner

Simple and Savory Winter Fish Stew (see the recipe in appendix
A)

Green salad tossed with extra-virgin olive oil and lemon juice to
taste

8 ounces water

2 high-quality Norwegian fish oil capsules

Bedtime

1 hard-boiled egg

3 cherry tomatoes

3 macadamia nuts

8 ounces water

Important Note: If you are taking the neuropeptide supplement, it is
now time to cut your dose. Starting with Day 13, take one neuropeptide supplement once daily or once every other day with breakfast.

DAY 13. Saturday

Start the day with 1 teaspoon peptide functional food powder
mixed with 6 ounces water or Maitake Fraction-D or Fraction-SX.
Exercise for the day.
After cleansing, apply neuropeptide cream to face and throat.

Breakfast

Omelet made with 2 whole eggs and 2 egg whites, fresh herbs,
and chopped scallions or chives

Yogurt or kefir smoothie—mix in blender 6 ounces unsweetened
kefir, ¼ cup mixed berries, 1 teaspoon ground flaxseed, and
1 serving açaí

3 almonds
8 ounces green tea or water

Supplements: Daily supplement regimen, 2 high-quality Norwegian fish oil capsules, 1 neuropeptide supplement

Lunch

Salmon Salad (see the recipe in appendix A)
2-inch wedge cantaloupe
8 ounces water

Supplements: Daily supplement regimen, 2 high-quality Norwegian fish oil capsules

Snack

1 hard-boiled egg
1 apple
3 walnuts
8 ounces water

Dinner

Mediterranean Stuffed Peppers (see the recipe in appendix A)
Green salad tossed with extra-virgin olive oil and lemon juice to
    taste
8 ounces water
2 high-quality Norwegian fish oil capsules

Bedtime

½ cup cottage cheese topped with 1 tablespoon chopped
    pumpkin or sunflower seeds
1 kiwi fruit
8 ounces water

DAY 14. Sunday

Start the day with 1 teaspoon peptide functional food powder mixed with 6 ounces water or Maitake Fraction-D or Fraction-SX.
Exercise for the day: Relaxation.
After cleansing, apply neuropeptide cream to face and throat.

Breakfast
    2 slices turkey bacon
    2 soft-boiled eggs
    ½ cup Buckwheat Cereal (see the recipe in appendix A)
    8 ounces green tea or water

Supplements: Daily supplement regimen, 2 high-quality Norwegian fish oil capsules, 1 neuropeptide supplement

Lunch
    Caesar Salad with Grilled Chicken or Shrimp (see the recipe in
        appendix A)
    2-inch wedge cantaloupe

Supplements: Daily supplement regimen, 2 high-quality Norwegian fish oil capsules

Snack
    Yogurt or kefir smoothie—mix in blender 6 ounces unsweetened
        kefir, ¼ cup mixed berries, 1 teaspoon ground flaxseed, and 1
        serving açaí
    8 ounces water

Dinner
    Chicken-Walnut Salad with White Beans and Artichokes (see the
        recipe in appendix A)
    1 pear
    8 ounces water
    2 high-quality Norwegian fish oil capsules

Bedtime
    1 ounce sliced turkey breast
    3 olives
    3 cherry tomatoes
    8 ounces water

WEEK THREE

DAY 15. Monday

Start the day with 1 teaspoon peptide functional food powder mixed with 6 ounces water or Maitake Fraction-D or Fraction-SX. Exercise for the day.
After cleansing, apply neuropeptide cream to face and throat.

Breakfast
    1 soft-boiled egg
    ½ cup cottage cheese topped with 1 tablespoon ground flaxseed
    ⅛–¼ cup (measure before cooking) old-fashioned oatmeal with
        ½ teaspoon cinnamon
    ¼ cup berries
    8 ounces green tea or water

Supplements: Daily supplement regimen, 2 high-quality Norwegian fish oil capsules, 1 neuropeptide supplement

Lunch
    ¾ cup Ginger Chicken or Tofu Salad (see the recipe in appendix
        A)
    1 kiwi fruit
    8 ounces water

Supplements: Daily supplement regimen, 2 high-quality Norwegian fish oil capsules

Snack
 6 ounces plain yogurt or kefir mixed with 1 package pure açaí
   pulp
 3 almonds
 8 ounces water

Dinner
 Hazelnut-Encrusted Wild Salmon Fillets on a Bed of Wilted
   Greens (see the recipe in appendix A)
 2-inch wedge cantaloupe
 8 ounces water
 2 high-quality Norwegian fish oil capsules

Bedtime
 1 hard-boiled egg
 1 apple
 3 walnuts
 8 ounces water

DAY 16. Tuesday

Start the day with 1 teaspoon peptide functional food powder
mixed with 6 ounces water or Maitake Fraction-D or Fraction-SX.
 After cleansing, apply neuropeptide cream to face and throat.

Breakfast
 Omelet made with 2 whole eggs, 2 egg whites, and fresh herbs
 Yogurt or kefir smoothie—6 ounces plain yogurt, 1 tablespoon
   ground flaxseed, ¼ cup mixed berries, and 1 serving açaí
 8 ounces green tea or water

Supplements: Daily supplement regimen, 2 high-quality Norwegian fish oil capsules, 1 neuropeptide supplement

Lunch

> Greek Salad Topped with Grilled Chicken, Salmon, Shrimp, or
> Tofu (see the recipe in appendix A)
> 1 apple
> 8 ounces water

Supplements: Daily supplement regimen, 2 high-quality Norwegian fish oil capsules

Snack

> ½ cup cottage cheese topped with 1 tablespoon ground
> flaxseed
> 1 pear
> 8 ounces water

Dinner

> 1 bowl Rich Lentil and Turkey Sausage Soup (see the recipe in
> appendix A)
> 1 cup dark green leafy salad with 3–6 ounces grilled chicken
> dressed with olive oil and lemon juice to taste and ½ cup
> sprouts
> 8 ounces water
> 2 high-quality Norwegian fish oil capsules

Bedtime

> 1–2 ounces sliced roast turkey or chicken breast
> 1 tablespoon raw pumpkin seeds
> 2-inch wedge honeydew melon
> 8 ounces water

DAY 17. Wednesday

Start the day with 1 teaspoon peptide functional food powder mixed with 6 ounces water or Maitake Fraction-D or Fraction-SX.
Exercise for the day.
After cleansing, apply neuropeptide cream to face and throat.

Breakfast
4–8 ounces grilled or smoked salmon
½ cup cooked barley with ½ teaspoon cinnamon topped with 1
    tablespoon berries
8 ounces green tea or water

Supplements: Daily supplement regimen, 2 high-quality Norwegian fish oil capsules, 1 neuropeptide supplement

Lunch
Jumbo Shrimp Cocktail (see the recipe in appendix A)
½ avocado
1 apple
8 ounces water

Supplements: Daily supplement regimen, 2 high-quality Norwegian fish oil capsules

Snack
6 ounces plain yogurt mixed with 1 package pure açaí
1 tablespoon sunflower seeds
8 ounces water

Dinner
Chicken Almond Ding (see the recipe in appendix A)
½ cup fruit salad with mixed berries, kiwi, and pear
8 ounces water
2 high-quality Norwegian fish oil capsules

Bedtime
¼ cup Hummus (see the recipe in appendix A)
1 celery stalk
8 ounces water

DAY 18. Thursday

Start the day with 1 teaspoon peptide functional food powder mixed with 6 ounces water or Maitake Fraction-D or Fraction-SX. Exercise for the day.
After cleansing, apply neuropeptide cream to face and throat.

Breakfast
Omelet made with 2 whole eggs, 2 egg whites, ½ ounce
  crumbled feta, and ¼ teaspoon dried or fresh dill weed
2-inch wedge cantaloupe
8 ounces green tea or water

Supplements: Daily supplement regimen, 2 high-quality Norwegian fish oil capsules, 1 neuropeptide supplement

Lunch
Crab or Lobster Cocktail (see the recipe in
  appendix A)
Green salad dressed with extra-virgin olive oil and lemon juice
  to taste
1 pear
8 ounces water

Supplements: Daily supplement regimen, 2 high-quality Norwegian fish oil capsules

Snack
Kefir smoothie—mix in blender 6 ounces unsweetened kefir, ¼ cup
  mixed berries, 1 teaspoon ground flaxseed, and 1 serving açaí
8 ounces water

Dinner
Curried Chicken or Tofu (see the recipe in appendix A) served
  on ½ cup cooked barley
Cool and Creamy Cucumber Salad (see the recipe in appendix A)
8 ounces water
2 high-quality Norwegian fish oil capsules

Bedtime

1–2 ounces sliced turkey or chicken breast

¼ cup cherries

3 almonds

8 ounces water

DAY 19. Friday

Start the day with 1 teaspoon peptide functional food powder mixed with 6 ounces water or Maitake Fraction-D or Fraction-SX.

Exercise for the day.

After cleansing, apply neuropeptide cream to face and throat.

Breakfast

1 soft-boiled egg

2 slices turkey bacon

Yogurt or kefir smoothie—mix in blender 6 ounces plain yogurt or kefir, ¼ cup mixed berries, and 1 serving açaí

8 ounces green tea or water

Supplements: Daily supplement regimen, 2 high-quality Norwegian fish oil capsules, 1 neuropeptide supplement

Lunch

Chicken, Turkey, or Tofu Salad Wrap (see the recipe in appendix A)

8 ounces water

Supplements: Daily supplement regimen, 2 high-quality Norwegian fish oil capsules

Snack

1 hard-boiled egg

3 cherry tomatoes

3 olives

8 ounces water

Dinner

Salmon Teriyaki (can also be made with chicken breast or tofu—
see the recipe in appendix A)

½ cup steamed asparagus

½ cup lentils

8 ounces water

2 high-quality Norwegian fish oil capsules

Bedtime

½ cup cottage cheese

1 tablespoon chopped pumpkin seeds

8 ounces water

DAY 20. Saturday

Start the day with 1 teaspoon peptide functional food powder
mixed with 6 ounces water or Maitake Fraction-D or Fraction-SX.
Exercise for the day.
After cleansing, apply neuropeptide cream to face and throat.

Breakfast

2 slices Canadian or turkey bacon

½ cup cottage cheese

½ cup Buckwheat Cereal (see the recipe in appendix A)

1 kiwi fruit

8 ounces green tea or water

Supplements: Daily supplement regimen, 2 high-quality Norwegian fish oil capsules, 1 neuropeptide supplement

Lunch

½ cup Hummus (see the recipe in appendix A)

4–6 ounces broiled chicken, salmon, or tofu

2 celery stalks

1 apple

Supplements: Daily supplement regimen, 2 high-quality Norwegian fish oil capsules

Snack
    Yogurt smoothie—mix in blender 6 ounces plain yogurt and 1
       serving açaí
    3 walnuts
    8 ounces water

Dinner
    Grilled Indian Chicken (see the recipe in appendix A)
    ½ cup Baked Barley (see the recipe in appendix A)
    2-inch wedge cantaloupe
    8 ounces water
    2 high-quality Norwegian fish oil capsules

Bedtime
    1–2 ounces sliced turkey or chicken breast
    ¼ cup pumpkin seeds
    ½ cup cherries
    8 ounces water

DAY 21. Sunday

Start the day with 1 teaspoon peptide functional food powder mixed with 6 ounces water or Maitake Fraction-D or Fraction-SX.
Exercise for the day: Relaxation.
After cleansing, apply neuropeptide cream to face and throat.

Breakfast
    3–6 ounces broiled or smoked salmon
    ⅛–¼ cup (measure before cooking) old-fashioned oatmeal with
       ½ teaspoon cinnamon
    1 kiwi fruit
    8 ounces green tea or water

Supplements: Daily supplement regimen, 2 high-quality Norwegian fish oil capsules, 1 neuropeptide supplement

Lunch

Turkey Burger (see the recipe in appendix A)
Green salad dressed with extra-virgin olive oil and lemon juice
   to taste
½ cup berries
8 ounces water

Supplements: Daily supplement regimen, 2 high-quality Norwegian fish oil capsules

Snack

½ cup cottage cheese topped with 1 tablespoon ground flaxseed
1 apple
8 ounces water

Dinner

Savory Halibut with Braised Red Peppers and Leeks (see the
   recipe in appendix A)
½ cup Buckwheat Pilaf (see the recipe in appendix A)
8 ounces water
2 high-quality Norwegian fish oil capsules

Bedtime

1–2 ounces sliced turkey or chicken breast
3 olives
3 strawberries
8 ounces water

WEEK FOUR

DAY 22. Monday

Start the day with 1 teaspoon peptide functional food powder mixed with 6 ounces water or Maitake Fraction-D or Fraction-SX. Exercise for the day.
After cleansing, apply neuropeptide cream to face and throat.

Breakfast
Omelet made with 2 whole eggs, 2 egg whites, fresh herbs, and
  chopped chives or scallions
Yogurt or kefir smoothie—mix in blender 6 ounces unsweetened
  kefir, ¼ cup mixed berries, 1 teaspoon ground flaxseed, and 1
  serving açaí
8 ounces green tea or water

Supplements: Daily supplement regimen, 2 high-quality Norwegian fish oil capsules, 1 neuropeptide supplement

Lunch
Jumbo Shrimp, Crab, or Lobster Cocktail (see the recipe in
  appendix A)
Green salad dressed with extra-virgin olive oil and lemon juice
  to taste, garnished with ½ avocado
1 pear
8 ounces water

Supplements: Daily supplement regimen, 2 high-quality Norwegian fish oil capsules

Snack
½ cup cottage cheese topped with 1 tablespoon chopped
  sunflower or pumpkin seeds
1 apple
8 ounces water

Dinner

Lemon Chicken (see the recipe in appendix A)

Saffron-Scented Oat Pilaf with Parsley (see the recipe in appendix A)

Mixed fruit plate with thinly sliced melon, kiwi, and apple

8 ounces water

2 high-quality Norwegian fish oil capsules

Bedtime

1–2 ounces sliced turkey or chicken breast

3 almonds

¼ cup blueberries

8 ounces water

DAY 23. Tuesday

Start the day with 1 teaspoon peptide functional food powder mixed with 6 ounces water or Maitake Fraction-D or Fraction-SX.

Exercise for the day.

After cleansing, apply neuropeptide cream to face and throat.

Breakfast

Omelet made with 2 whole eggs and 2 egg whites filled with ½ cup sautéed onions and mushrooms

2-inch wedge honeydew melon

8 ounces green tea or water

Supplements: Daily supplement regimen, 2 high-quality Norwegian fish oil capsules, 1 neuropeptide supplement

Lunch

Hearty Chicken Soup (see the recipe in appendix A)

1 pear

8 ounces water

Supplements: Daily supplement regimen, 2 high-quality Norwegian fish oil capsules

Snack

1–2 ounces turkey breast
3 walnuts
1 apple
8 ounces water

Dinner

Baked Scrod with Tomato-Basil Sauce (see the recipe in
   appendix A)
Spinach with Garlic and Ginger (see the recipe in appendix A)
½ cup Baked Barley (see the recipe in appendix A)
¼ cup berries
8 ounces water
2 high-quality Norwegian fish oil capsules

Bedtime

½ cup cottage cheese topped with 1 tablespoon ground
   flaxseed
¼ cup cherries
8 ounces water

DAY 24. Wednesday

Start the day with 1 teaspoon peptide functional food powder
mixed with 6 ounces water or Maitake Fraction-D or Fraction-SX.
Exercise for the day.
After cleansing, apply neuropeptide cream to face and throat.

Breakfast

3–6 ounces grilled salmon fillet or lox
Yogurt or kefir smoothie—mix in blender 6 ounces unsweetened
   kefir, ¼ cup mixed berries, and 1 serving açaí

3 macadamia nuts
8 ounces green tea or water

Supplements: Daily supplement regimen, 2 high-quality Norwegian fish oil capsules, 1 neuropeptide supplement

Lunch

Chicken, Turkey, or Tofu Salad Wrap (see the recipe in appendix A)
Large green salad with sliced tomatoes
2-inch wedge cantaloupe
8 ounces water

Supplements: Daily supplement regimen, 2 high-quality Norwegian fish oil capsules

Snack

½ cup Hummus (see the recipe in appendix A)
2 celery stalks
3 almonds
8 ounces water

Dinner

Curried Shrimp (see the recipe in appendix A)
½ cup cooked whole oats or barley—cooked in the same manner as brown rice
1 cup salad made with mixed baby greens and ½ avocado, dressed with extra-virgin olive oil and lemon juice to taste
8 ounces water
2 high-quality Norwegian fish oil capsules

Bedtime

1–2 ounces sliced chicken or turkey breast
¼ cup pumpkin seeds
1 apple
8 ounces water

DAY 25. Thursday

Start the day with 1 teaspoon peptide functional food powder mixed with 6 ounces water or Maitake Fraction-D or Fraction-SX. Exercise for the day.

After cleansing, apply neuropeptide cream to face and throat.

Breakfast
Omelet made with 2 eggs and 2 egg whites, fresh herbs, and
   1 ounce feta cheese
⅛–¼ cup (measure before cooking) old-fashioned oatmeal
   topped with 1 tablespoon chopped pumpkin seeds
1 kiwi fruit
8 ounces green tea or water

Supplements: Daily supplement regimen, 2 high-quality Norwegian fish oil capsules, 1 neuropeptide supplement

Lunch
Salmon Burger on a Bed of Baby Greens (see the recipe in
   appendix A)
1 apple
8 ounces water

Supplements: Daily supplement regimen, 2 high-quality Norwegian fish oil capsules

Snack
Yogurt or kefir smoothie—mix in blender 6 ounces unsweetened
   kefir, ¼ cup mixed berries, 1 teaspoon ground flaxseed, and 1
   serving açaí
8 ounces green tea or water

Dinner
Two-Bean Turkey or Tofu Chili (see the recipe in appendix A)
Green salad dressed with extra-virgin olive oil and lemon juice
   to taste

1 pear

8 ounces water

2 high-quality Norwegian fish oil capsules

Bedtime

½ cup cottage cheese topped with 1 teaspoon flaxseed

¼ cup berries

8 ounces water

DAY 26. Friday

Start the day with 1 teaspoon peptide functional food powder mixed with 6 ounces water or Maitake Fraction-D or Fraction-SX.

Exercise for the day.

After cleansing, apply neuropeptide cream to face and throat.

Breakfast

2 links turkey or tofu sausage

2 soft-boiled eggs

½ cup cooked barley topped with 1 tablespoon yogurt and
    ¼ cup berries

8 ounces green tea or water

Supplements: Daily supplement regimen, 2 high-quality Norwegian fish oil capsules, 1 neuropeptide supplement

Lunch

Mediterranean Turkey Soup (see the recipe in appendix A)

3 walnuts

2-inch wedge cantaloupe

Supplements: Daily supplement regimen, 2 high-quality Norwegian fish oil capsules

Snack

    Yogurt or kefir smoothie—mix in blender 6 ounces unsweetened
        kefir, ¼ cup mixed berries, 1 teaspoon ground flaxseed, and 1
        serving açaí

    8 ounces water

Dinner

    Simple and Savory Winter Fish Stew (see the recipe in appendix
        A)

    Green salad tossed with extra-virgin olive oil and lemon juice to
        taste

    8 ounces water

    2 high-quality Norwegian fish oil capsules

Bedtime

    1 hard-boiled egg

    3 cherry tomatoes

    3 macadamia nuts

    8 ounces water

DAY 27. Saturday

Start the day with 1 teaspoon peptide functional food powder
mixed with 6 ounces water or Maitake Fraction-D or Fraction-SX.
    Exercise for the day.
    After cleansing, apply neuropeptide cream to face and throat.

Breakfast

    Omelet made with 2 whole eggs and 2 egg whites, fresh herbs,
        and chopped scallions or chives

    Yogurt or kefir smoothie—mix in blender 6 ounces unsweetened
        kefir, ¼ cup mixed berries, 1 teaspoon ground flaxseed, and 1
        serving açaí

    3 almonds

    8 ounces green tea or water

Supplements: Daily supplement regimen, 2 high-quality Norwegian fish oil capsules, 1 neuropeptide supplement

Lunch
Salmon Salad (see the recipe in appendix A)
2-inch wedge cantaloupe
8 ounces water

Supplements: Daily supplement regimen, 2 high-quality Norwegian fish oil capsules

Snack
1 hard-boiled egg
1 apple
3 walnuts
8 ounces water

Dinner
Mediterranean Stuffed Peppers (see the recipe in appendix A)
Green salad tossed with extra-virgin olive oil and lemon juice to
    taste
8 ounces water
2 high-quality Norwegian fish oil capsules

Bedtime
½ cup cottage cheese topped with 1 tablespoon chopped
    pumpkin or sunflower seeds
1 kiwi fruit
8 ounces water

DAY 28. Sunday

Start the day with 1 teaspoon peptide functional food powder
mixed with 6 ounces water or Maitake Fraction-D or Fraction-SX.
    Exercise for the day: Relaxation.
    After cleansing, apply neuropeptide cream to face and throat.

Breakfast

2 slices turkey bacon

2 soft-boiled eggs

½ cup Buckwheat Cereal (see the recipe in appendix A)

8 ounces green tea or water

Supplements: Daily supplement regimen, 2 high-quality Norwegian fish oil capsules, 1 neuropeptide supplement

Lunch

Caesar Salad with Grilled Chicken or Shrimp (see the recipe in appendix A)

2-inch wedge cantaloupe

Supplements: Daily supplement regimen, 2 high-quality Norwegian fish oil capsules

Snack

Yogurt or kefir smoothie—mix in blender 6 ounces unsweetened kefir, ¼ cup mixed berries, 1 teaspoon ground flaxseed, and 1 serving açaí

8 ounces water

Dinner

Chicken-Walnut Salad with White Beans and Artichokes (see the recipe in appendix A)

1 pear

8 ounces water

2 high-quality Norwegian fish oil capsules

Bedtime

1 ounce sliced turkey breast

3 olives

3 cherry tomatoes

8 ounces water

I hope that you follow my program and find that it has helped change your life. My patients tell me that this is what happened to them, and I know it will happen for you, too. This is the pathway to a new and better life; may you walk it with joy and enjoy the reward it can bring.

Recipes for the 28-Day Perricone Program

THESE RECIPES USE MANY OF THE RAINBOW FOODS, superfoods, and herbs and spices featured in chapters 3, 4, and 5. They're designed to be nutrient-dense and full of antioxidants. They're easy to follow, and taste great.

Breakfast

Buckwheat Cereal

Makes 2 servings

2 cups water
1 cup buckwheat groats
1 apple, cored and chopped
¼ cup sunflower seeds
1 teaspoon cinnamon
¼ cup yogurt

Bring 2 cups of water to a boil. Add the buckwheat. Return to a boil. Stir once.

Add the apple, seeds, and cinnamon.

Turn the heat to low and cook, uncovered, for 20 minutes or until grain is cooked. Serve hot topped with yogurt.

Lunch

Hummus

Makes a great dip with celery stalks and other raw vegetables. This is a grea
lunch dish or snack, with protein, fiber, antioxidants, and calcium. Adapte
from The Whole Food Bible.

Makes about 2½ cups

1½ cups cooked or canned chickpeas plus ½ cup bean liquid (use
    water if you don't have any bean liquid)
3 cloves garlic, peeled
¼ cup sesame tahini (ground sesame seeds, available at health foo
    stores and in the natural food section of supermarkets)
2 tablespoons extra-virgin olive oil
Juice of 1 lemon
1 teaspoon sea salt
Lettuce leaves
Cayenne pepper or paprika

Place the chickpeas and garlic in a blender or food processor. Puree
until the beans begin to break down.

Add a quarter to half of the reserved liquid or water (depending
on the desired consistency), the tahini, olive oil, lemon juice, and salt.
Continue to puree until all the ingredients are well blended and the
mixture has a smooth consistency. Chill for at least 2 hours.

Serve on a bed of lettuce. Garnish with a sprinkle of cayenne
pepper or paprika.

Chicken, Turkey, or Tofu Salad Wrap

Serves 2

For the wrap

1½ cups cubed cooked chicken or turkey breast or firm tofu
½ stalk celery, chopped
1 small apple, cored and chopped
4 walnuts, chopped
1 tablespoon fresh lemon juice
½ cup alfalfa or broccoli sprouts
2 large, washed cabbage leaves

Mix all the ingredients (except the cabbage leaves) together in a small bowl. Divide the mixture into two portions and spread each leaf with half. Roll up the cabbage leaf and tuck in the ends as if making an egg roll.

For the dressing

1 cup yogurt
1 tablespoon lemon juice
1 teaspoon chopped fresh parsley
1 teaspoon chopped fresh or dried dill

Mix the yogurt, lemon juice, and herbs into a dressing and serve on the side.

Salmon Burgers on a Bed of Baby Greens

This is a quick and delicious lunch or dinner recipe.

Makes 3 burgers

1 can (14.75 ounces) wild Alaskan salmon
3 scallions, minced
1 tablespoon finely grated peeled fresh ginger
1 large egg white
1 tablespoon soy sauce
1 tablespoon olive oil
1½ cups baby greens

Drain the salmon and then stir it together with the scallions and ginger in a large glass or ceramic bowl until well combined.

Beat together the egg white and soy sauce in a small bowl and stir into the salmon mixture; form into 3 (½-inch-thick) patties.

Heat the olive oil in a 12-inch skillet over medium heat. Add the patties and cook, carefully turning once, until golden brown and cooked through, approximately 6 to 7 minutes.

Arrange greens on plates. Place hot burgers on the greens and serve immediately.

Salmon Salad

Makes 2 servings

1 pound cooked salmon, cubed, or 1 can (15 ounces) salmon, drained
Juice of 1 large lemon
1 cup cooked or canned white beans, drained
⅓ cup extra-virgin olive oil
Chopped fresh tarragon leaves from several sprigs
1 cup cherry tomatoes, halved
¼ cup chopped scallions
¼ cup minced fresh basil leaves
¼ cup minced fresh parsley leaves
Salt and freshly ground black pepper, to taste
4 cups romaine lettuce torn into bite-sized pieces

Gently toss the salmon with the lemon juice, beans, and olive oil. Add the remaining ingredients and continue to toss until the dressing is evenly distributed.

Ginger Chicken or Tofu Salad

Adapted from The Whole Food Bible.

Serves 2

2 cups chopped cooked chicken breast or firm tofu
¼ cup chopped red onion
½ stalk celery
1 teaspoon sunflower seeds
¼ teaspoon finely minced fresh ginger
1½ tablespoons extra-virgin olive oil
2 tablespoons fresh lemon juice
Romaine lettuce

Toss all the ingredients together until fully coated with olive oil and lemon juice. Serve on a bed of romaine lettuce.

Turkey Burgers

This recipe can be used for burgers or cooked in a loaf pan like a traditional meat loaf. Adapted from The Whole Food Bible.

Makes 4 burgers or 1 loaf

1½ pounds ground organic free-range turkey
¼ cup minced onion
¾ cup coarsely ground oatmeal (put in a blender and pulse until the oatmeal is the consistency of bread crumbs)
1 egg
¼ cup minced celery
¼ cup milk, soy milk, or stock
1 teaspoon sea salt
1 garlic clove, minced
3 tablespoons chopped fresh parsley

Mix all the ingredients well. Form into 1-inch-thick patties and place in a lightly oiled skillet. Cook the burgers over medium heat for about 5 minutes, or until browned and crispy. Flip the burgers carefully and cook for 5 minutes longer, or until golden brown and a thermometer inserted in the center registers 165° and the meat is no longer pink. Serve the burgers hot.

If you're making a loaf, preheat the oven to 350°F. Form the mixture into a loaf and pack into a lightly oiled 8 x 4-inch baking pan. Bake for approximately 45 minutes, or until the loaf begins to pull away from the pan.

Jumbo Shrimp, Crab, or Lobster Cocktail

Many of today's finer supermarkets will cook the shrimp, crab, or lobster for you, making this simple yet delicious meal even easier.

Arrange 4 to 6 large shrimp or 4 to 6 ounces of lump crabmeat or lobster meat chunks in a small bowl. Garnish with lemon wedges. Serve with cocktail sauce.

For the cocktail sauce

¼ cup ketchup (use Westbrae unsweetened ketchup, available at natural food stores or in the natural food section of the supermarket)
1–1½ tablespoons fresh lemon juice
3 tablespoons drained bottled horseradish, or to taste
¼ teaspoon Tabasco

Blend all the ingredients together with a fork. Serve chilled.

Mediterranean Turkey Soup

Makes 4 servings

1 tablespoon olive oil
1 green or red bell pepper, diced
1 yellow onion, chopped
2 ribs celery, chopped
3 large cloves garlic, chopped
1 tablespoon dried basil
2 teaspoons fennel seeds
¼ teaspoon dried crushed red pepper
6 cups low-salt chicken broth
1 can (28 ounces) plum tomatoes, chopped and drained
1 can (15 ounces) white beans
1½ pounds diced cooked turkey
Grated Parmesan or Romano cheese
Salt and pepper

Heat the oil in a heavy large saucepan over medium heat. Add the bell pepper, onion, celery, garlic, basil, fennel seeds, and crushed red pepper. Sauté for about 10 minutes or until tender.

Add the broth and tomatoes. Cover the pan and simmer for 10 minutes.

Add the beans and turkey and cook until heated through, about 1 minute.

Garnish each soup bowl with 1 tablespoon of cheese, adding salt and pepper to taste.

Hearty Chicken Soup

Makes 4 servings

6 cups low-salt chicken broth
1 cup uncooked whole oats or barley
2 tablespoons chopped fresh thyme or 2 teaspoons dried, crumbled
1 tablespoon olive oil
1 onion, chopped
2 celery stalks, chopped
2 scallions, thinly sliced
3 large cloves garlic, chopped
1½ pounds diced cooked chicken breast
Salt and pepper
Chopped fresh parsley

In a large stockpot or Dutch oven, bring the chicken broth to a boil. Add the oats or barley and thyme. Return the soup to a boil.

Reduce the heat to medium and simmer the soup, uncovered, until the oats are tender, stirring occasionally, about 30 minutes.

In a large skillet, heat 1 tablespoon of olive oil. Sauté the onion, celery, scallions, and garlic over medium heat until translucent. Transfer the vegetables to the chicken broth.

Add the chicken and simmer until heated through, thinning with additional broth if desired. Season with salt and pepper. Garnish with parsley and serve.

Greek Salad Topped with Grilled Chicken, Salmon, Shrimp, or Tofu

Makes 2 generous servings

2 tablespoons extra-virgin olive oil
2 teaspoons fresh lemon juice
1 clove garlic, minced
1 cup baby spinach leaves or romaine lettuce torn into bite-sized pieces
1 small green bell pepper, chopped
½ cucumber, chopped
½ red onion, sliced
1 cup cherry tomatoes, halved
⅓ cup Greek or kalamata olives
2 teaspoons finely chopped fresh oregano
3 tablespoons chopped fresh Italian parsley
1 (6-ounce) piece feta, quartered
½ cup chickpeas
Freshly ground black pepper, to taste
8–12 ounces grilled chicken, salmon, shrimp, or tofu

Whisk the olive oil, lemon juice, and garlic together in a small bowl. Set aside.

Combine the rest of the ingredients in a large wooden salad bowl. Add the dressing and gently toss until all ingredients are coated.

Caesar Salad with Grilled Chicken or Shrimp

Makes 2 servings

2 cups romaine lettuce torn into bite-sized pieces
1 large clove garlic, minced
¼ cup extra-virgin olive oil
Salt and freshly ground pepper, to taste
½ teaspoon Worcestershire sauce
Juice of 1 lemon
¼ cup freshly grated pecorino Romano cheese
8–12 ounces grilled chicken breast, cut into strips, or 8 jumbo
  shrimp

Wash and dry the lettuce.

With a wooden spoon, mash the garlic in a large wooden salad bowl. Add the lettuce and olive oil and toss until the lettuce is thoroughly coated with the oil. Add the seasonings, Worcestershire sauce, and lemon juice and continue to toss. Add the grated cheese and toss gently until evenly distributed over the lettuce.

Arrange the chicken or shrimp on top of the salad.

Dinner

SEAFOOD

Savory Halibut with Braised Red Peppers and Leeks

This is a simple dish to make, but it will taste as if you've spent hours on it. Cod, sole, or another firm fish can be substituted for the halibut. This dish can be cooked on the grill or under a broiler. Serve with a grain such as barley or oats to soak up the marinade. Adapted from The Whole Food Bible.

Makes 4 generous servings

1½ pounds halibut
2 red bell peppers, cored, seeded, and cut into thin strips
3 medium leeks, white part only, sliced thin and washed well

For the marinade

3 tablespoons extra-virgin olive oil
2 tablespoons low-sodium tamari (soy sauce available at health food
   stores)
2 tablespoons fresh lemon juice
2 tablespoons dry white wine
2 cloves garlic, minced
2 quarter-sized pieces fresh gingerroot, peeled and minced

Wash the halibut and pat dry. Combine the marinade ingredients and place the fish and marinade in a glass or ceramic dish. Marinate for 1 hour in the refrigerator, turning several times.

Light the grill (if you're using charcoal or wood as opposed to gas) 45 minutes prior to cooking, or preheat the broiler 15 minutes before cooking.

Remove the fish from the marinade and set aside. Put the marinade into a large skillet and heat. Add the red pepper and leeks and sauté over medium heat for 15 minutes, or until tender. Do not brown.

After the vegetables have sautéed for 5 minutes, place the halibut over white coals, or under the broiler 4 to 6 inches from the heat. Cook for 4 to 5 minutes on each side or until the flesh is opaque throughout and flakes easily.

Place the fish on serving plates and top with the braised red peppers and leeks.

Curried Shrimp

Curry, ginger, and garlic combine in this easy recipe to create a delicious meal. Serve with a side dish of whole oats or barley prepared as you would brown rice. Adapted from The Whole Food Bible.

Makes 4 servings

1½ pounds shrimp, shelled and deveined
Juice of 1 lime
3 tablespoons olive oil
3 small onions, coarsely chopped
2 cloves garlic, minced
2 quarter-sized pieces fresh gingerroot, peeled and minced
1–2 tablespoons curry powder, to taste
3 large tomatoes, chopped, plus 1 cup tomato juice, or 1 undrained
    can (14 ounces) tomatoes

Sprinkle the shrimp (or chicken or tofu) with the lime juice and set aside.

Heat the oil in a large skillet. Add the onions, garlic, and ginger. Cook over medium heat, stirring often, until the onions are translucent, about 5 minutes. Do not brown.

Add the curry powder, stir well, and continue to sauté the mixture for 3 more minutes, stirring frequently. Add the tomatoes and juice. Stir, cover, and let simmer for 15 minutes, stirring occasionally.

Uncover the skillet and add the shrimp. Stir well and cook over medium heat for 3 to 5 minutes, until the shrimp turn pink. Serve immediately.

Salmon Teriyaki

The teriyaki sauce in this recipe can also be used with chicken or tofu. If you are using wooden skewers, be sure to soak them in water first to keep them from scorching. Adapted from The Whole Food Bible.

Makes 4 servings

For the teriyaki sauce

¼ cup reduced-sodium tamari
¼ cup dry sherry
1 tablespoon sesame oil
1 tablespoon freshly grated gingerroot
2 garlic cloves, put through a garlic press

For the fish

2 pounds wild Alaskan salmon steaks or fillets
Lemon wedges

Combine the ingredients for the sauce.

Place the fish in a glass or ceramic dish, pour the marinade over, and marinate in the refrigerator for 2 hours.

Light a fire in the grill or preheat the broiler. Remove the fish from the marinade and transfer to a plate. Grill the fish over white coals (or under the broiler), basting with the marinade, for 3 to 4 minutes. Turn and grill, basting again, for another 3 to 4 minutes. Do not overcook.

Any leftover marinade can be reheated and served with the fish. Garnish with lemon wedges.

Hazelnut-Encrusted Wild Salmon Fillets
on a Bed of Wilted Greens

Almonds or sunflower seeds may also be used in place of hazelnuts. Adapted from The Whole Food Bible.

Makes 4 servings

½ cup almonds
¼ cup chopped fresh parsley
1 tablespoon grated organic lemon zest (use organic lemons to
    avoid nonorganic lemon rind, which is treated with fungicide)
Dash of sea salt and fresh pepper
4 skinless salmon fillets, 6 ounces each
2 tablespoons olive oil
4 cups mixed organic baby greens (arugula, mesclun, spinach, etc.)
Lemon wedges

Grind the almonds in a coffee grinder or food processor—do not overgrind and turn into a paste. Mix the almonds, parsley, lemon zest, salt, and pepper on a plate.

Dry the salmon; dredge the fillets on both sides in the almond mixture.

Heat the oil in a large skillet over medium heat. Add the salmon and cook for about 5 minutes on each side, making sure that the salmon is cooked through.

Arrange 1 cup of greens per plate. Transfer the hot salmon fillets to the plates. Garnish with lemon wedges and serve immediately.

Simple and Savory Winter Fish Stew

This Mediterranean-style fish stew uses lots of tomatoes and garlic. A variety of different types of seafood can be used, all with great success, although my favorite choice is the wild Alaskan salmon. Serve with a crisp green salad. Adapted from The Whole Food Bible.

Makes 4 large servings

1 can (28 ounces) plum tomatoes plus juice
2 tablespoons extra-virgin olive oil
2 onions, chopped
5 cloves garlic, chopped
2 cups dry white wine*
3 tablespoons chopped fresh basil, oregano, and thyme
4 cups water
2 cups fish stock or clam juice
A few threads of saffron
1 can (15 ounces) organic Great Northern or other white beans
2 pounds salmon, halibut, scrod, or cusk, cut into bite-sized
    cubes
Sea salt and freshly ground pepper, to taste
Dash of cayenne pepper, to taste

Drain and chop the tomatoes, reserving the juice, and set aside.

In a large soup pot, heat the olive oil and gently sauté the onions and garlic over medium heat until translucent, about 5 minutes. Do not brown. Add the wine, tomatoes, tomato juice, and herbs, and continue sautéing for another 5 minutes.

Add the water and stock or clam juice and bring to a boil. Add the saffron and gently simmer for 5 to 8 minutes. Add the beans and fish and gently simmer, covered, for 10 minutes. Season with salt, pepper, and cayenne to taste, and serve.

*Once the wine boils, most of its alcohol content evaporates.

Baked Scrod with Tomato–Basil Sauce

This recipe couldn't be simpler or more delicious. Baked barley is an excellent accompaniment, along with a crisp green salad. Adapted from The Whole Food Bible.

Makes 4 servings

2 tablespoons extra-virgin olive oil
2 pounds scrod, cut into 4 serving pieces

For the sauce

2 cups chopped fresh basil
3 large cloves garlic, chopped
½ teaspoon sea salt
¼ teaspoon ground pepper
⅛ teaspoon cayenne pepper
2 tablespoons extra-virgin olive oil
2 tablespoons red wine vinegar
2 cups minced plum tomatoes

Preheat the oven to 400°F.

Sprinkle 2 tablespoons olive oil over the bottom of an ovenproof casserole large enough to hold the fish. Place the fish on top of the oil.

Place the basil, garlic, salt, pepper, cayenne, 2 tablespoons olive oil, and vinegar in a blender or food processor. Puree for 10 seconds. Add the tomatoes and blend until the tomatoes are chopped but not pureed.

Spoon the sauce over the fish, cover, and bake for 15 to 20 minutes, or until the flesh is opaque and flakes easily.

POULTRY

Lemon Chicken

Adapted from The Whole Food Bible.

Makes 4 generous servings

1 teaspoon sea salt
/4 teaspoon ground pepper
/2 cup ground sunflower seeds or walnuts
2 pounds free-range, all-natural chicken breasts, halved, skinned,
 boned, and pounded to ¼ inch thick
3 tablespoons olive oil
¼ cup dry white wine
¼ cup fresh lemon juice
1 tablespoon butter
2 tablespoons minced fresh parsley
1 lemon, thinly sliced

Mix the salt and pepper into the ground seeds or nuts. Dredge the
chicken pieces in the mixture. Shake off the excess and set aside.

In a large skillet, heat the oil over medium heat. Sauté the chicken
breasts until lightly browned, about 3 minutes per side. Remove from
the pan and place on paper towels, turning once to absorb excess oil.

Combine the wine and lemon juice and pour into the skillet.
Bring to a boil and scrape down any bits of chicken stuck to the sides
of the pan. Add the chicken pieces and simmer in the liquid for 5
minutes. Remove to a heated platter.

Raise the heat to high, bring the liquid to a boil, and reduce the
liquid to ¼ cup. Whisk in the butter and pour over the chicken. Garnish with parsley and lemon slices.

Chicken Almond Ding

Don't let the list of ingredients intimidate you; stir-frying is a quick and easy way to put together a meal. Serve over cooked whole oats or barley. Adapted from The Whole Food Bible.

Makes 4 generous servings

For the marinade

3 tablespoons low-sodium tamari
3 tablespoons dry sherry
3 cloves garlic, minced
2 tablespoons minced fresh ginger
1 tablespoon extra-virgin olive oil
2 pounds chicken breasts, skinned, boned, and cut into ½-inch strips

In a medium glass or ceramic bowl, combine all the ingredients for the marinade. Add the chicken and let sit at room temperature for at least 15 minutes and up to an hour.

For the stir-fry

3 tablespoons extra-virgin olive oil
3 cups broccoli florets
¼ pound mushrooms, cleaned and cut into ¼-inch slices
3 celery stalks, cut into ¼-inch diagonal slices
⅛ pound pea pods, trimmed
3 scallions, thinly sliced (use both the bulb and the green leaves)
1 cup lightly toasted almonds*
1 teaspoon Asian (toasted) sesame oil (available in natural food stores)

Heat a wok or large skillet. Add 1 tablespoon of the olive oil. Stir-fry the broccoli over medium heat until it turns a bright color, 3 to 4 minutes. Remove from the pan and set aside.

Reheat the wok. Add 1 tablespoon of the olive oil. Stir-fry the mushrooms, celery, and pea pods for 2 to 3 minutes. Remove from the wok and set aside.

Reheat the wok. Add the remaining tablespoon of the olive oil. Remove the chicken from the marinade with a slotted spoon, add to the wok, and stir-fry until the chicken is opaque throughout, about 5 minutes. Add all the vegetables along with the scallions and almonds, and stir to mix well. Remove from the heat. Sprinkle with the toasted sesame oil. Serve immediately over cooked whole oats or barley.

*To toast the almonds, place in a preheated 350°F oven for 8 to 10 minutes, or until lightly browned.

Grilled Indian Chicken

Serve with a crisp salad and your favorite rice dish, substituting barley or oats for the rice. Adapted from The Whole Food Bible.

Makes 4 servings

2 pounds skinless, boneless chicken breasts

For the marinade

1 cup plain yogurt
1 teaspoon turmeric
1 teaspoon paprika
¼ teaspoon cardamom
1 tablespoon freshly squeezed lemon juice
2 tablespoons freshly squeezed lime juice
2 tablespoons extra-virgin olive oil
1 tablespoon finely grated ginger
4 large cloves garlic, minced
½ teaspoon ground cumin
4 scallions, greens included, minced
¼ teaspoon sea salt
White or red pepper to taste
Lemon or lime wedges for garnish

Cut the skinless chicken breasts into 1-inch pieces. Place in a medium bowl.

In another bowl, combine the yogurt, turmeric, paprika, cardamom, lemon and lime juices, olive oil, ginger, garlic, cumin, scallions, salt, and pepper. Pour the marinade over the cubed chicken and mix well with your hands to coat the pieces evenly. Marinate in the refrigerator for 2 hours.

Thread the chicken onto skewers and cook over a medium-hot fire for 5 to 7 minutes, turning frequently. Baste the chicken with leftover marinade after turning. Serve with the lemon or lime wedges.

Rich Lentil and Turkey Sausage Soup

This soup is rich enough to be served as a main dinner course. It has protein and fiber, and is rich in antioxidants. Adapted from The Whole Food Bible.

Makes 6 servings

2 cups lentils
8–10 cups vegetable broth or water
2 tablespoons extra-virgin olive oil
4 cloves garlic, minced
1 large onion, chopped
2 celery stalks, chopped
1 pound all-natural turkey or chicken sausage
2 tomatoes, peeled, seeded, and chopped (or 1 can, 15 ounces, chopped or crushed tomatoes)
1 teaspoon turmeric, or to taste
1 teaspoon ground cumin
Leaves from 1 sprig fresh thyme, or ½ teaspoon dried thyme
Pinch of dried red pepper flakes
Sea salt, to taste
Plain yogurt, for garnish
½ cup chopped fresh parsley (flat-leafed, if available), for garnish

Wash and pick over the lentils (to make sure there are no stones) and bring to a boil in the broth or water in a large soup pot. Lower the heat and simmer for 10 minutes.

Meanwhile, heat the olive oil in a large skillet. Sauté the garlic, onion, celery, and sausage for 5 minutes over medium heat. Add the tomatoes and sauté for another 5 minutes.

Add the vegetable-sausage mixture and seasonings to the lentils. Simmer for 20 to 30 minutes, or until the lentils are tender but not mushy. Serve with a dollop of plain yogurt and chopped parsley for garnish.

Curried Chicken or Tofu

Curry, ginger, and garlic combine in this easy recipe to create a delicious meal. Serve with a side dish of whole oats or barley prepared as you would brown rice. Adapted from The Whole Food Bible.

Makes 4 servings

1½ pounds skinless, boneless chicken breasts or firm tofu, cubed
Juice of 1 lime
3 tablespoons olive oil
3 small onions, coarsely chopped
2 cloves garlic, minced
2 quarter-sized pieces fresh gingerroot, peeled and minced
1–2 tablespoons curry powder, to taste
3 large tomatoes, chopped, plus 1 cup tomato juice, or 1 undrained
 can (14 ounces)

Sprinkle the chicken or tofu with the lime juice and set aside.

Heat the oil in a large skillet. Add the onions, garlic, and ginger. Cook over medium heat, stirring often, until the onions are translucent, about 5 minutes. Do not brown.

Add the curry powder, stir well, and continue to sauté the mixture for 3 more minutes, stirring frequently. Add the tomatoes and juice. Stir, cover, and let simmer for 15 minutes, stirring occasionally.

Uncover the skillet and add the chicken or tofu. Stir well and cook over medium heat for 10 to 15 minutes or until the chicken is thoroughly cooked; if you're using tofu, 3 to 5 minutes should be enough cooking time. Serve immediately.

Mediterranean Stuffed Peppers

Either red or green bell peppers work in this recipe, the red being sweeter. Adapted from The Whole Food Bible.

Makes 3 main-course servings, or 6 side-dish servings

2 tablespoons extra-virgin olive oil
1 large onion, minced
1½ pounds ground turkey
1 cup whole barley
1¾ cups water
6 medium red or green bell peppers
½ cup sunflower seeds
¼ cup freshly grated pecorino Romano cheese
¼ cup fresh mint, minced
¼ cup fresh parsley, minced
¼ cup fresh lemon juice
¼ cup dry white wine
½ teaspoon ground cinnamon
Sea salt and freshly ground pepper, to taste

Preheat the oven to 350°F.

In a 2- or 3-quart saucepan, heat the olive oil and sauté the onion and ground turkey over medium heat for about 10 minutes. Add the barley and sauté, stirring often, for a few minutes. Add the water, bring to a boil, reduce the heat, and simmer for 45 minutes or until all the water is absorbed.

Bring a large pot of water to a boil. Meanwhile, cut off the tops of the peppers with care—they will be used later. Gently remove the cores and seeds to create an empty cavity. Blanch the peppers in the boiling water for 5 minutes. Remove from the water and place upside down on paper towels to drain.

Roast the sunflower seeds on a baking sheet in the preheated oven for about 5 minutes, shaking the pan often. Remove and set aside, leaving the oven on for the peppers.

When the barley is done, toss it with the sunflower seeds, cheese, herbs, lemon juice, wine, cinnamon, salt, and pepper in a large bowl. Mix well and adjust the seasonings to taste. Stuff the peppers with the mixture, put the tops back on, and place the peppers in a baking dish just large enough to hold them upright. Bake for 25 to 30 minutes, or until the barley mixture is heated through. Serve immediately.

Two-Bean Turkey or Tofu Chili

Use canned beans for a quick meal on the table. Mix and match varieties—kidney, pinto, black, and so on. Adapted from The Whole Food Bible.

Makes 6 servings

2 tablespoons extra-virgin olive oil
1 large Spanish onion, chopped
3 cloves garlic, minced
1 red and 1 yellow pepper (or 2 red peppers), chopped
2 pounds freshly ground turkey or firm tofu, cubed
1 tablespoon ground cumin
2 tablespoons chili powder
2¼ cups cooked kidney or pinto beans, drained, or 1 can
    (15 ounces)
2¼ cups cooked white beans, drained, or 1 can (15 ounces)
1 can (28 ounces) plum tomatoes, chopped, with liquid
1 tablespoon balsamic vinegar
Tabasco sauce or cayenne pepper, to taste
Chopped black olives, scallions, and 1 tablespoon grated Parmesan
    or Romano cheese per serving

In a 5- to 6-quart soup pot, heat the olive oil and sauté the onion, garlic, and peppers for 10 minutes over medium heat. Add the turkey or tofu and sauté for another 5 minutes. Add the cumin and chili powder and cook for 5 minutes more.

Add the cooked beans, chopped plum tomatoes and their liquid, and balsamic vinegar. Cook, covered, for 15 minutes.

Add Tabasco or cayenne to taste and cook, covered, for another 15 minutes. Serve piping hot garnished with chopped olives, scallions, and grated cheese.

Chicken-Walnut Salad with White Beans and Artichokes

Makes 4 servings

2 pounds cooked skinless and boneless chicken breasts, cubed
¼ cup thinly sliced red onion
3 stalks celery, sliced
½ cup walnuts, chopped
1 cup artichoke hearts, halved
10 cherry tomatoes, halved
2 cups mixed baby greens
3 tablespoons chopped fresh parsley
3 tablespoons extra-virgin olive oil
⅓ cup fresh lemon juice
⅓ cup freshly grated pecorino Romano cheese
Salt and pepper, to taste
1 cup cooked or canned white or garbanzo beans

In a large wooden salad bowl, gently toss the chicken, onion, celery, walnuts, artichoke hearts, tomatoes, greens, and parsley. Add the olive oil and continue to toss until ingredients are lightly coated.

Add lemon juice and toss lightly. Add the grated cheese, salt, pepper, and beans, and continue to toss lightly until the cheese is evenly distributed.

Garnish with lemon wedges and serve.

Side Dishes

Spinach with Garlic and Ginger

Adapted from The Whole Food Bible.

Makes 4 servings

1½ pounds spinach
2 tablespoons extra-virgin olive oil
3 cloves garlic, minced
1 tablespoon minced, peeled fresh ginger
⅛ teaspoon dried red pepper flakes
¼ cup water
Toasted sesame seeds, for garnish*

Wash the spinach thoroughly.

Heat the oil in a large skillet. Add the garlic, ginger, and red pepper flakes. Cook over medium heat for 30 seconds, stirring often. Add the spinach and stir for 1 minute to blend. Add the water and continue to sauté, stirring, until the spinach is completely wilted.

Remove the spinach to a platter with a slotted spoon. Garnish with sesame seeds.

---

*To toast sesame seeds, stir them in a dry pan over medium heat until lightly browned.

Baked Barley

Barley is an ancient and healthy grain. It takes well to baking, remaining firm and chewy. Baked barley can be enjoyed with seafood and chicken dishes, and the leftovers can be turned into a hearty grain salad. Adapted from The Whole Food Bible.

Makes 6 side-dish servings

½ cup sunflower seeds
3 shallots, peeled and minced
1 onion, minced
1 leek, well cleaned and thinly sliced
3 tablespoons extra-virgin olive oil
½ pound mushrooms, sliced
3 celery stalks, chopped
1 cup barley
1 teaspoon dried thyme
1 teaspoon dried rosemary
1 teaspoon dried marjoram
2 tablespoons low-sodium all-natural tamari
3 cups boiling vegetable stock or water

Preheat the oven to 350°F. Toast the sunflower seeds in the oven for about 7 minutes, or until lightly browned; remove from the oven, leaving it at 350°.

In a large skillet, sauté the shallots, onion, and leek in the olive oil for 5 minutes over medium heat. Add the mushrooms, celery, sunflower seeds, barley, herbs, and tamari and continue sautéing for 5 more minutes, stirring frequently.

Add the vegetable stock or water to the barley mixture. Bring to a boil and transfer the mixture to a casserole dish. Bake, covered, for 1¼ hours.

Saffron-Scented Oat Pilaf with Parsley

Adapted from The Whole Food Bible.

Makes 4 servings

2 cups water or broth
⅛ teaspoon saffron, crushed
2 tablespoons extra-virgin olive oil
1 shallot or large clove garlic, minced
1 medium yellow onion, diced
1 cup whole oat groats (they look like brown rice—available at
   natural food stores)
½ cup fresh parsley
Leaves from 2 stalks fresh rosemary, or 1 teaspoon dried rosemary
4 tablespoons Parmesan or Romano cheese (for superior flavor,
   use imported cheese and grate it yourself)

Boil ½ cup of the water or broth and pour it over the saffron. Set
aside.

Heat the oil in a large saucepan. Sauté the shallot and onion over
medium heat for about 5 minutes. Add the oats and stir to coat all the
grains. Cook over medium heat for about 5 minutes, stirring frequently.

Add the remaining 1½ cups of water or broth, then add the saffron
mixture and bring to a boil. Reduce the heat to a simmer and cook,
covered, for about 45 minutes, or until all the water is absorbed.

Remove the cover, fluff the oats with a fork, fold in the herbs, and
serve immediately. Top each serving with 1 tablespoon grated
Parmesan or Romano cheese.

Buckwheat Pilaf

Makes 4 servings

2 tablespoons extra-virgin olive oil
1 onion, chopped
1 cup uncooked whole buckwheat
3½ cups chicken stock
¼ teaspoon oregano
1 tablespoon grated orange rind (use organic orange)
⅓ cup finely chopped pecans (optional)
Salt and pepper, to taste
2 tablespoons chopped parsley
¼ cup freshly grated pecorino Romano cheese

Heat the olive oil in large saucepan and sauté the onion until translu-cent. Add the buckwheat. Stir well. Add the chicken stock, cover, and cook for approximately 20 minutes or until all the liquid is absorbed.

Add the oregano, orange rind, pecans, and salt and pepper. Stir and serve, topping each serving with parsley and cheese.

Cool and Creamy Cucumber Salad

This salad is cool and refreshing and makes a great accompaniment to a spicy dish. Adapted from The Whole Foods Bible.

Makes 4 salad servings

1½ cups yogurt
3 cucumbers, peeled, seeded, and diced fine
1 clove garlic, minced
1 tablespoon extra-virgin olive oil
2 tablespoons fresh lemon juice
Dash of sea salt and pepper, to taste

Mix all the ingredients well and chill in the refrigerator for 2 hours.

Resource Guide

Topical Peptide-Neuropeptide Products
(Anti-Inflammatory/Anti-Aging)

N. V. Perricone, M.D., Ltd., at 888-823-7837 or
www.nvperriconemd.com
N. V. Perricone, M.D., Ltd., Flagship Store at 791 Madison Avenue
(at 67th Street), New York, NY
Nordstrom
Sephora.com
Selected Saks
Selected Neiman Marcus
Henri Bendel
Clyde's on Madison (926 Madison Avenue at 74th Street,
New York, NY)
Bloomingdales

Topical Peptide Products (Not Neuropeptides)

cannot vouch for any of the products listed below, because I have
not tested them. Please note that if the stated content is "pentapep-
ides," these are not neuropeptides. Pentapeptides *do not* demonstrate
he efficacy of the sophisticated neuropeptides, each of which has to
be synthesized on an individual basis. These pentapeptides cost dollars
per pound and simply cannot deliver the level of efficacy that the
neuropeptides do, whose cost may exceed thirteen thousand dollars
per pound!

- Neova Copper Peptide
- StriVectin-SD
- Olay Regenerist
- Philosophy When Hope Is Not Enough
- Pentapeptide-SF Eye Contour Serum
- DDF Wrinkle Relax
- Desert Essence Age Reversal Face Serum
- Desert Essence Age Reversal Face Cream

Topical Anti-Aging, Anti-Inflammatory
Skin Products with Alpha Lipoic Acid and DMAE

- N.V. Perricone, M.D., Ltd., at 888-823-7837 or www.nvperriconemd.com
- N.V. Perricone, M.D., Ltd., Flagship Store at 791 Madison Avenue (at 67th Street), New York, NY
- Nordstrom
- Sephora.com
- Selected Saks
- Selected Neiman Marcus (store locator at www.neimanmarcus.com/store/info/index.jhtml)
- Henri Bendel
- Clyde's on Madison (926 Madison Avenue at 74th Street, New York, NY)
- Bloomingdales

Polysaccharide Peptide Food Products
(Anti-Inflammatory/Anti-Aging)

- N.V. Perricone, M.D., Ltd., at 888-823-7837 or www.nvperriconemd.com
- N.V. Perricone, M.D., Ltd., Flagship Store at 791 Madison Avenue (at 67th Street), New York, NY

Maitake D-Fraction and SX-Fraction Extract

Maitake Products, Inc., at 800-747-7418 or www.maitake.com
* www.gnc.com
  www.americannutrition.com
* www.wellfx.com
* www.vitamindiscountwarehouse.com
* www.vitacost.com

Peptide Supplements

N.V. Perricone, M.D., Ltd., at 888-823-7837 or
www.nvperriconemd.com

Rainbow Foods

AÇAÍ (AMAZONIAN FRUIT HIGH IN ANTIOXIDANTS)

Açaí fruit has more antioxidants than wild blueberries, pomegranates, or red wine, along with essential omegas (healthy fats), amino acids, calcium, and fiber. Sambazon is the sole U.S. source of açaí beverages, at www.sambazon.com. Sambazon brand açaí beverages can also be found nationwide at Whole Foods Market and Wild Oats stores, and in some health food stores and juice bars. Sambazon—whose name is an acronym for "saving and managing the Brazilian Amazon"—supports indigenous economies through responsible extraction and sustainable development, harvesting fruit as a renewable resource of the rain forest rather than harvesting the forest itself.

POMEGRANATE JUICE AND CONCENTRATE (EXTREMELY HIGH IN ANTIOXIDANTS)

* POM Wonderful at 310-966-5800 or www.pomwonderful.com
* Also available at supermarkets and natural food stores.

WILD ALASKAN SALMON/TUNA/HALIBUT

Vital Choice Seafood at www.vitalchoice.com or 800-608-4825
Wild Alaskan salmon has a healthier fatty acid profile (less saturated
fat, a higher ratio of omega-3 fatty acids to saturated fats) compared
with noticeably "greasy" farmed salmon. Vital Choice Seafood products (salmon, tuna, and halibut) are caught at sea, flash-frozen immediately, packed in dry ice, and delivered via FedEx or UPS at
affordable prices. In 2000, wild Alaskan salmon was the first fishery
certified sustainable by the Marine Stewardship Council.

FLAVORFUL, HEALTHFUL RECIPES

The Whole Food Bible, by Christopher Kilham, available at
www.amazon.com and www.innertraditions.com.

HEALTH EDUCATION INFORMATION

These Web sites offer interesting information on the topics of nutrition, natural healing, addiction, and holistic health:

* www.tuberose.com
* www.doitnow.com

ORGANIC BERRIES

* Diamond Organics, Inc., sells certified-organic berries (in season,
  May through October) direct to consumers. Go to www
  .diamondorganics.com/fruit.html#summer or
  call 888-ORGANIC (888-674-2642).
* Vital Choice Seafood sells wild organic blueberries, at www
  .vitalchoice.com or 800-608-4825.

ORGANIC RAINBOW FRUITS AND VEGETABLES

* Diamond Organics, Inc., sells certified-organic fruits and
  vegetables direct to consumers. Go to www.diamondorganics

.com/vegetables.html and www.diamondorganics.com/fruit.html
or call 800-434-4246.

Ten Superfoods

AÇAÍ (AMAZONIAN FRUIT HIGH IN ANTIOXIDANTS)

ee the entry under Rainbow Foods.

ALLIUM VEGETABLES
(ONIONS, GARLIC, SCALLIONS, SHALLOTS, LEEKS)

Diamond Organics, Inc., sells certified-organic Allium family vegetables direct to consumers. Go to www.diamondorganics.com/
rootsandtubers.html or call 800-434-4246.

BARLEY AND BUCKWHEAT

Diamond Organics, Inc., sells certified-organic barley and buckwheat direct to consumers. Go to www.diamondorganics.com/
wholegrains.html or call 800-434-4246.

GREEN FOODS: BARLEY GRASS, WHEAT GRASS, SPIRULINA,
CHLORELLA, BLUE-GREEN ALGAE (BGA)

- Barley grass products at
  www.mothernature.com/shop/sections/index.cfm/s/99378
- Wheat grass products at
  www.mothernature.com/shop/sections/index.cfm/s/99383
- Chlorella products at
  www.mothernature.com/shop/sections/index.cfm/s/99395
- Blue-green algae (BGA) products at
  www.mothernature.com/shop/sections/index.cfm/s/99394
- Mixed green food products at
  www.mothernature.com/shop/sections/index.cfm/s/99379

- Green Foods Corporation at www.greenfoods.com/home.html. Retail and Web outlets at www.greenfoods.com/products/where_to_buy.html
- Spirulina at www.mothernature.com/shop/sections/index.cfm/s/99399 or www.earthrise.com

BEANS AND LENTILS

- Westbrae Natural markets certified-organic beans, including rare heirloom varieties, nationwide. Go to www.westbrae.com/products/index.html or call 800-434-4246.

HOT PEPPERS (CHILIES)

- Diamond Organics, Inc., sells certified-organic chili peppers direct to consumers. Go to www.diamondorganics.com/vegetables.html#peppers or call 888-674-2642.

NUTS AND SEEDS

- Diamond Organics, Inc., markets a wide variety of organic foods, including certified-organic nuts and seeds. Go to www.diamondorganics.com/dryfruitandnuts.html or call 888-674-2642.
- Jaffee Bros. Natural Foods, founded in 1948, specializes in organic fruits, nuts, and seeds. Go to organicfruitsandnuts.com/default.asp or call 760-749-1133.

KEFIR AND YOGURT

- Helios Nutrition is a small organic dairy in Sauk Centre, Minnesota, that makes several flavors of organic kefir with added FOS (prebiotic polysaccharide). Locate retail outlets at 888-3-HELIOS or www.heliosnutrition.com/html/where_to_buy.html.

- Stonyfield Farm yogurt is available at many food markets. See the store locator at www.stonyfield.com/StoreLocator/.
- Horizon Organic yogurt is available at many food markets. See the store locator at www.horizonorganic.com/findingproducts/index.html.
- Diamond Organics, Inc., sells organic yogurt direct to consumers at www.diamondorganics.com/dairy.html#straus or 800-434-4246.
- Lifeway Kefir can be found at www.lifeway.com, at Lifeway Foods, Inc., 6431 West Oakton Avenue, Morton Grove, IL 60053, 847-967-1010, and at Royal Baltic, 9829 Ditmas Avenue, Brooklyn, NY 11236, 718-385-7152.

SPROUTS

- The International Sprout Growers Association (ISGA) at www.isga-sprouts.org is the professional association of sprout growers and companies, which supplies products and services to the sprout industry. Visit its Web site for outstanding information, recipes, and health notes.
- "Sproutman" Steve Meyerowitz is one of the world's leading proponents of do-it-yourself sprouting. His excellent, highly informative Web site will get you started growing your own windowsill garden twelve months a year. You can reach Steve Meyerowitz and Sproutman Publications at 413-528-5200, www.sproutman.com, or P.O. Box 1100, Great Barrington, MA 01230.

Spices of Life

New Chapter, Inc., markets high-potency ginger and turmeric extract supplements (Gingerforce and Turmericforce), as well as formulas that combine various anti-inflammatory herbs, such as Zyflamend, which has been used in successful prostate cancer inhibition test-tube studies at Columbia University.

New Chapter extracts contain an unusually broad spectrum of each plant's active constituents because they employ the high-tech "supercritical" carbon dioxide method as well as standard water and alcohol extraction. New Chapter products are described at www.new-chapter.com/product/supercritical.lasso, and retail sources can be found at 800-543-7279 or www.new-chapter.com/buy/index.html.

Nutritional Supplements

WEIGHT MANAGEMENT PROGRAM SUPPLEMENTS

Weight management program supplements formulated by N.V. Perricone, M.D., are available from:

- N.V. Perricone, M.D., Ltd., at 888-823-7837 or www.nvperriconemd.com
- N.V. Perricone, M.D., Ltd., Flagship Store at 791 Madison Avenue (at 67th Street), New York, NY
- Nordstrom
- Sephora
- Selected Saks
- Selected Neiman Marcus

ANTI-AGING, ANTI-INFLAMMATORY SUPPLEMENTS

Total Skin and Body nutritional supplements, formulated by N.V. Perricone, M.D., are available from:

- N.V. Perricone, M.D., Ltd., at 888-823-7837 or www.nvperriconemd.com
- N.V. Perricone, M.D., Ltd., Flagship Store at 791 Madison Avenue (at 67th Street), New York, NY
- Nordstrom
- Sephora.com
- Selected Saks
- Selected Neiman Marcus

ANTI-AGING VITAMIN-MINERAL-NUTRIENT SUPPLEMENTS

N.V. Perricone, M.D., Ltd., at 888-823-7837 or
www.nvperriconemd.com
N.V. Perricone, M.D., Ltd., Flagship Store at 791 Madison Avenue
(at 67th Street), New York, NY
Optimum Health International at 800-228-1507 or
www.opthealth.com
Life Extension Foundation at 800-544-4440 or www.lef.org

HIGH-QUALITY FISH OIL CAPSULES

N.V. Perricone, M.D., Ltd., at 888-823-7837 or
www.nvperriconemd.com
- N.V. Perricone, M.D., Ltd., Flagship Store at 791 Madison Avenue
(at 67th Street), New York, NY
- Vital Choice Seafood at 800-608-4825 or www.vitalchoice.com.
- Optimum Health International at 800-228-1507 or
www.opthealth.com

BENFOTIAMINE SUPPLEMENTS

Benfotiamine is a synthetic variant of vitamin B_1 with unique anti-
aging effects.

- www.nvperriconemd.com
- Benfotiamine.net at www.benfotiamine.net
- iHerb.com at www.iherb.com/benfotiamine.html

ANTI-ACNE, ANTI-INFLAMMATORY SUPPLEMENTS

The SkinClear Nutritional Support System is formulated by N.V.
Perricone, M.D., and is available from:

- N.V. Perricone, M.D., Ltd., at 888-823-7837 or www.nvperriconemd.com
- Nordstrom
- Sephora
- Selected Saks
- Selected Neiman Marcus

OPC GRAPE SEED EXTRACT SUPPLEMENTS

Flavay brand OPC supplements are manufactured to the specifications of Jacques Masquelier, Ph.D., the discoverer OPCs and holder of international patents. Accordingly, Flavay brand OPC supplements match the specifications of the OPC-rich grape seed extracts used in most of the laboratory tests and clinical trials conducted to date. Order Flavay products at 800-200-1203, 775-787-6737, or www.healthyalternatives.com/order.html.

BERRY EXTRACT ANTHOCYANIN SUPPLEMENTS

InterHealth USA markets OptiBerry, a blend of wild blueberry, strawberry, cranberry, wild bilberry, elderberry, and raspberry extracts that contains extraordinarily high guaranteed levels of biologically active anthocyanins. Products containing OptiBerry can be found at www.interhealthusa.com/faqs/optiberry_faqs.aspx#wherecanibuyit.

RESVERATROL (HUZHANG EXTRACT) SUPPLEMENTS

InterHealth USA markets Protykin, a 200:1 standardized extract of huzhang *(Polygonum cuspidatum),* which is rich in resveratrol—one of the antioxidants that give grapes and red wine exceptional heart-health and anti-cancer properties. Products containing Protykin can be found at www.interhealthusa.com/faqs/protykin_faqs.aspx#wherecanibuyit.

References

Chapters 1 and 2

Arion VY, Zimina IV, Lopuchin YM. Contemporary views on the nature and clinical application of thymus preparations. Russ J Immunol. 1997 Dec;2(3-4):157-66.

Association of Early Childhood Educators, Ontario, Canada. The importance of touch for children. Posted August 1997 at http://collections.ic.gc.ca/child/docs/00000949.htm.

Balasubramaniam A. Clinical potentials of neuropeptide Y family of hormones. Am J Surg. 2002 Apr;183(4):430-4. Review.

Ben-Efraim S, Keisari Y, Ophir R, Pecht M, Trainin N, Burstein Y. Immunopotentiating and immunotherapeutic effects of thymic hormones and factors with special emphasis on thymic humoral factor THF-gamma2. Crit Rev Immunol. 1999;19(4):261-84. Review.

Berczi I, Chalmers IM, Nagy E, Warrington RJ. The immune effects of neuropeptides. Baillieres Clin Rheumatol. 1996 May;10(2):227-57. Review.

Black PH. Stress and the inflammatory response: a review of neurogenic inflammation. Brain Behav Immun. 2002 Dec;16(6):622-53. Review.

Bodey B. Thymic hormones in cancer diagnostics and treatment. Expert Opin Biol Ther. 2001 Jan;1(1):93-107. Review.

Bodey B, Bodey B Jr, Siegel SE, Kaiser HE. Review of thymic hormones in cancer diagnosis and treatment. Int J Immunopharmacol. 2000 Apr;22(4):261-73. Review.

Datar P, Srivastava S, Coutinho E, Govil G. Substance P: structure, function, and therapeutics. Curr Top Med Chem. 2004;4(1):75-103. Review.

Davis TP, Konings PN. Peptidases in the CNS: formation of biologically active, receptor-specific peptide fragments. Crit Rev Neurobiol. 1993;7(3-4):163-74. Review.

Friedman MJ. What might the psychobiology of posttraumatic stress disorder teach us about future approaches to pharmacotherapy? J Clin Psychiatry. 2000;61 Suppl 7:44-51. Review.

Frucht-Pery J, Feldman ST, Brown SI. The use of capsaicin in herpes zoster ophthalmicus neuralgia. Acta Ophthalmol Scand. 1997 Jun;75(3):311-3.

Galli L, de Martino M, Azzari C, Bernardini R, Cozza G, de Marco A, Lucarini D, Sabatini C, Vierucci A. [Preventive effect of thymomodulin in recurrent respiratory infections in children.] Pediatr Med Chir. 1990 May-Jun;12(3):229-32. Italian.

Gambert SR, Garthwaite TL, Pontzer CH, Cook EE, Tristani FE, Duthie EH, Martinson DR, Hagen TC, McCarty DJ. Running elevates plasma beta-endorphin immunoreactivity and ACTH in untrained human subjects. Proc Soc Exp Biol Med. 1981 Oct;168(1):1-4.

Geenen V, Kecha O, Brilot F, Hansenne I, Renard C, Martens H. Thymic T-cell tolerance of neuroendocrine functions: physiology and pathophysiology. Cell Mol Biol (Noisy-le-grand). 2001 Feb;47(1):179-88. Review.

Gianoulakis C. Implications of endogenous opioids and dopamine in alcoholism: human and basic science studies. Alcohol Alcohol Suppl. 1996 Mar;1:33-42. Review.

Goldstein AL, Badamchian M. Thymosins: chemistry and biological properties in health and disease. Expert Opin Biol Ther. 2004 Apr;4(4):559-73.

Goldstein AL, Schulof RS, Naylor PH, Hall NR. Thymosins and anti-thymosins: properties and clinical applications. Med Oncol Tumor Pharmacother. 1986;3(3-4):211-21. Review.

Goya RG, Console GM, Herenu CB, Brown OA, Rimoldi OJ. Thymus and aging: potential of gene therapy for restoration of endocrine thymic function in thymus-deficient animal models. Gerontology. 2002 Sep-Oct;48(5):325-8.

Gutzwiller JP, Degen L, Matzinger D, Prestin S, Beglinger C. Interaction between GLP-1 and CCK33 in inhibiting food intake and appetite in men. Am J Physiol Regul Integr Comp Physiol. 2004 Apr 22.

Hill AJ, Peikin SR, Ryan CA, Blundell JE. Oral administration of proteinase inhibitor II from potatoes reduces energy intake in man. Physiol Behav. 1990 Aug;48(2):241-6.

Holmes A, Heilig M, Rupniak NM, Steckler T, Griebel G. Neuropeptide systems as novel therapeutic targets for depression and anxiety disorders. Trends Pharmacol Sci. 2003 Nov;24(11):580-8.

Hughes J, Kosterlitz HW, Smith TW. The distribution of methionine-enkephalin and leucine-enkephalin in the brain and peripheral tissues. 1977. Br J Pharmacol. 1997 Feb;120 (Suppl 4):428-36, discussion 426-7.

Jessop DS, Harbuz MS, Lightman SL. CRH in chronic inflammatory stress. Peptides. 2001 May;22(5):803-7. Review.

Kastin AJ, Zadina JE, Olson RD, Banks WA. The history of neuropeptide research: version 5.a. Ann NY Acad Sci. 1996 Mar 22;780:1-18. Review.

Katsuno M, Aihara M, Kojima M, Osuna H, Hosoi J, Nakamura M, Toyoda M, Matsuda H, Ikezawa Z. Neuropeptide concentrations in the skin of a murine (NC/Nga mice) model of atopic dermatitis. J Dermatol Sci. 2003 Oct;33(1):55-65.

Khavinson VKh. Peptides and ageing. Neuroendocrinol Lett. 2002;23 Suppl 3:11-144. Review.

Khavinson VKh, Morozov VG. Peptides of pineal gland and thymus prolong human life. Neuroendocrinol Lett. 2003 Jun-Aug;24(3-4):233-40.

Komarcevic A. [The modern approach to wound treatment.] Med Pregl. 2000 Jul-

Aug;53(7-8):363-8. Review. Croatian.

Kosterlitz HW, Corbett AD, Paterson SJ. Opioid receptors and ligands. NIDA Res Monogr. 1989;95:159-66. Review.

Kouttab NM, Prada M, Cazzola P. Thymomodulin: biological properties and clinical applications. Med Oncol Tumor Pharmacother. 1989;6(1):5-9. Review.

Kramer MS, Winokur A, Kelsey J, Preskorn SH, Rothschild AJ, Snavely D, Ghosh K, Ball WA, Reines SA, Munjack D, Apter JT, Cunningham L, Kling M, Bari M, Getson A, Lee Y. Demonstration of the efficacy and safety of a novel Substance P (NK1) receptor antagonist in major depression. Neuropsychopharmacology. 2004 Feb;29(2):385-92.

Li L, Zhou JH, Xing ST, Chen ZR. [Effect of thymic factor D on lipid peroxide, glutathione, and membrane fluidity in liver of aged rats.] Zhongguo Yao Li Xue Bao. 1993 Jul;14(4):382-4. Chinese.

Low TL, Goldstein AL. Thymosins: structure, function and therapeutic applications. Thymus. 1984;6(1-2):27-42. Review.

Maiorano V, Chianese R, Fumarulo R, Costantino E, Contini M, Carnimeo R, Cazzola P. Thymomodulin increases the depressed production of superoxide anion by alveolar macrophages in patients with chronic bronchitis. Int J Tissue React. 1989; 11(1):21–5.

Martin-Du-Pan RC. [Thymic hormones. Neuroendocrine interactions and clinical use in congenital and acquired immune deficiencies.] Ann Endocrinol (Paris). 1984;45(6):355-68. Review. French.

Morgan CA 3rd, Wang S, Southwick SM, Rasmusson A, Hazlett G, Hauger RL, Charney DS. Plasma Neuropeptide-Y concentrations in humans exposed to military survival training. Biol Psychiatry. 2000 May 15;47(10):902-9.

Pacher P, Kecskemeti V. Trends in the development of new antidepressants. Is there a light at the end of the tunnel? Curr Med Chem. 2004 Apr;11(7):925-43.

Pacher P, Kohegyi E, Kecskemeti V, Furst S. Current trends in the development of new antidepressants. Curr Med Chem. 2001 Feb;8(2):89-100. Review.

Paez X, Hernandez L, Baptista T. [Advances in the molecular treatment of depression.] Rev Neurol. 2003 Sep 1-15;37(5):459-70. Review. Spanish.

Parker J. Do It Now Foundation. www.doitnow.org

Pert CB, Pasternak G, Snyder SH. Opiate agonists and antagonists discriminated by receptor binding in brain. Science. 1973 Dec 28;182(119):1359-61.

Rains C, Bryson HM. Topical capsaicin. A review of its pharmacological properties and therapeutic potential in post-herpetic neuralgia, diabetic neuropathy and osteoarthritis. Drugs Aging. 1995 Oct;7(4):317-28. Review.

Rasmusson AM, Hauger RL, Morgan CA, Bremner JD, Charney DS, Southwick SM. Low baseline and yohimbine-stimulated plasma Neuropeptide Y (NPY) levels in combat-related PTSD. Biol Psychiatry. 2000 Mar 15;47(6):526-39.

Schulof RS. Thymic peptide hormones: basic properties and clinical applications in cancer. Crit Rev Oncol Hematol. 1985;3(4):309-76. Review.

Silva AP, Cavadas C, Grouzmann E. Neuropeptide Y and its receptors as potential therapeutic drug targets. Clin Chim Acta. 2002 Dec;326(1-2):3-25. Review.

Tada H, Nakashima A, Awaya A, Fujisaki A, Inoue K, Kawamura K, Itoh K, Masuda H,

Suzuki T. Effects of thymic hormone on reactive oxygen species-scavengers and renal function in tacrolimus-induced nephrotoxicity. Life Sci. 2002 Jan 25;70(10):1213-23.

Toyoda M, Morohashi M. New aspects in acne inflammation. Dermatology. 2003;206(1):17-23. Review.

Toyoda M, Nakamura M, Makino T, Hino T, Kagoura M, Morohashi M. Nerve growth factor and Substance P are useful plasma markers of disease activity in atopic dermatitis. Br J Dermatol. 2002 Jul;147(1):71-9.

Toyoda M, Nakamura M, Morohashi M. Neuropeptides and sebaceous glands. Eur J Dermatol. 2002 Sep-Oct;12(5):422-7. Review.

Chapter 3

Aquaxan™ HD algal meal use in aquaculture diets: enhancing nutritional performance and pigmentation. Technical report 2102.001. [www.fda.gov/ohrms/dockets/dailys/00/jun00/061900/rpt0065_tab6.pdf]

Arab L, Steck S. Lycopene and cardiovascular disease. Am J Clin Nutr. 2000;71:1691S-1695S.

Atalay M, Gordillo G, Roy S, Rovin B, Bagchi D, Bagchi M, Sen CK. Anti-angiogenic property of edible berry in a model of hemangioma. FEBS Lett. 2003 Jun 5;544(1-3):252-7.

Aviram M. 11th Biennial Meeting of the Society for Free Radical Research International, Paris, 2002.

Aviram M, Dornfeld L. Pomegranate juice consumption inhibits serum angiotensin converting enzyme activity and reduces systolic blood pressure. Atherosclerosis. 2001 Sep;158(1):195-8.

Aviram M, Dornfeld L, Kaplan M, Coleman R, Gaitini D, Nitecki S, Hofman A, Rosenblat M, Volkova N, Presser D, Attias J, Hayek T, Fuhrman B. Pomegranate juice flavonoids inhibit low-density lipoprotein oxidation and cardiovascular diseases: studies in atherosclerotic mice and in humans. Drugs Exp Clin Res. 2002;28(2-3):49-62. Review.

Aviram M, Dornfeld L, Rosenblat M, Volkova N, Kaplan M, Coleman R, Hayek T, Presser D, Fuhrman B. Pomegranate juice consumption reduces oxidative stress, atherogenic modifications to LDL, and platelet aggregation: studies in humans and in atherosclerotic apolipoprotein E-deficient mice. Am J Clin Nutr. 2000 May;71(5):1062-76.

Bagchi D, Bagchi M, Stohs SJ, Das DK, Ray SD, Kuszynski CA, Joshi SS, Pruess HG. Free radicals and grape seed proanthocyanidin extract: importance in human health and disease prevention. Toxicology. 2000 Aug 7;148(2-3):187-97.

Bagchi D, Bagchi M, Stohs S, Ray SD, Sen CK, Preuss HG. Cellular protection with proanthocyanidins derived from grape seeds. Ann NY Acad Sci. 2002 May;957:260-70. Review.

Bagchi D, Sen CK, Bagchi M, Atalay M. Anti-angiogenic, antioxidant, and anti-carcinogenic properties of a novel anthocyanin-rich berry extract formula. Biochemistry (Mosc). 2004 Jan;69(1):75-80.

Bianchini F, Vainio H. Wine and resveratrol: mechanisms of cancer prevention? Eur J Cancer Prev. 2003 Oct;12(5):417-25. Review.

Block G, Patterson B, Subar A. Fruit, vegetables, and cancer prevention: a review of the epidemiological evidence. Nutr Cancer. 1992;18(1):1-29. Review.

Burros M. Farmed salmon looking less rosy. New York Times, May 28, 2003.

Caballero-George C, Vanderheyden PM, De Bruyne T, Shahat AA, Van den Heuvel H, Solis PN, Gupta MP, Claeys M, Pieters L, Vauquelin G, Vlietinck AJ. In vitro inhibition of [3H]-angiotensin II binding on the human AT1 receptor by proanthocyanidins from Guazuma ulmifolia bark. Planta Med. 2002 Dec;68(12):1066-71.

Cal C, Garban H, Jazirehi A, Yeh C, Mizutani Y, Bonavida B. Resveratrol and cancer: chemoprevention, apoptosis, and chemo-immunosensitizing activities. Curr Med Chem Anti-Canc Agents. 2003 Mar;3(2):77-93. Review.

Calixto JB, Yunes RA. Natural bradykinin antagonists. Mem Inst Oswaldo Cruz. 1991;86 Suppl 2:195-202. Review.

Cao G, Russell RM, Lischner N, Prior RL. Serum antioxidant capacity is increased by consumption of strawberries, spinach, red wine or vitamin C in elderly women. J Nutr. 1998 Dec;128(12):2383-90.

Cao G, Shukitt-Hale B, Bickford PC, Joseph JA, McEwen J, Prior RL. Hyperoxia-induced changes in antioxidant capacity and the effect of dietary antioxidants. J Appl Physiol. 1999 Jun;86(6):1817-22.

Carson C, Lee S, De Paola C, et al. Antioxidant intake and cataract in the Melbourne Visual Impairment Project [abstract]. Am J Epidemiol. 1994;139 (Suppl 11):A65.

Dauer A, Hensel A, Lhoste E, Knasmuller S, Mersch-Sundermann V. Genotoxic and antigenotoxic effects of catechin and tannins from the bark of Hamamelis virginiana L. in metabolically competent, human hepatoma cells (Hep G2) using single cell gel elec-trophoresis. Phytochemistry. 2003 May;63(2):199-207.

Durak I, Avci A, Kacmaz M, Buyukkocak S, Cimen MY, Elgun S, Ozturk HS. Comparison of antioxidant potentials of red wine, white wine, grape juice and alcohol. Curr Med Res Opin. 1999;15(4):316-20.

Fahey JW, Zhang Y, Talalay P. Broccoli sprouts: an exceptionally rich source of inducers of enzymes that protect against chemical carcinogens. Proc Natl Acad Sci USA. 1997 Sep 16;94(19):10367-72.

Fisher ND, Hughes M, Gerhard-Herman M, Hollenberg NK. Flavanol-rich cocoa induces nitric-oxide-dependent vasodilation in healthy humans. J Hypertens. 2003 Dec;21(12):2281-6.

Flagg EW, Coates RJ, Greenberg RS. Epidemiologic studies of antioxidants and cancer in humans. J Am Coll Nutr. 1995;14:419-27.

Frances FJ. Pigments and other colorants. In: Food chemistry, 2nd edition. Fennema OR, ed. New York, Marcel Dekker, Inc., 1985.

Freedman JE, Parker C 3rd, Li L, Perlman JA, Frei B, Ivanov V, Deak LR, Iafrati MD, Folts JD. Select flavonoids and whole juice from purple grapes inhibit platelet function and enhance nitric oxide release. Circulation. 2001;103:2792-8.

Frieling UM, Schaumberg DA, Kupper TS, et al. A randomized, 12-year primary-prevention trial of beta carotene supplementation for nonmelanoma skin cancer in the Physicians' Health Study. Arch Dermatol. 2000;136:179-84.

Galli RL, Shukitt-Hale B, Youdim KA, Joseph JA. Fruit polyphenolics and brain aging: nutritional interventions targeting age-related neuronal and behavioral deficits. Ann NY Acad Sci. 2002 Apr;959:128-32. Review.

Gil MI, Tomas-Barberan FA, Hess-Pierce B, Holcroft DM, Kader AA. Antioxidant activity of pomegranate juice and its relationship with phenolic composition and processing. J Agric Food Chem. 2000 Oct;48(10):4581-9.

Giovannucci E. Tomatoes, tomato-based products, lycopene, and cancer: review of the epidemiologic literature. J Natl Cancer Inst. 1999;91:317-31.

Goldberg J, Flowerdew G, Smith E, et al. Factors associated with age-related macular degeneration. An analysis of data from the first National Health and Nutrition Examination Survey. Am J Epidemiol. 1988;128:700-10.

Gorman C, Park A. The fires within. Time. February 23, 2004.

Hackett AM. In: Plant flavonoids in biology and medicine: biochemical pharmacological and structure activity relationships. Cody V, Middleton EJ, Harborne JB, eds. New York, Liss 1986, 177-94.

Han B, Jaurequi J, Tang BW, Nimni ME. Proanthocyanidin: a natural crosslinking reagent for stabilizing collagen matrices. J Biomed Mater Res. 2003 Apr 1;65A(1):118-24.

Hennekens CH, Buring JE, Manson JE, et al. Lack of effect of long-term supplementation with beta carotene on the incidence of malignant neoplasms and cardiovascular disease. N Engl J Med. 1996;334:1145-9.

Holick CN, Michaud DS, Stolzenberg-Solomon R, Mayne ST, Pietinen P, Taylor PR, Virtamo J, Albanes D. Dietary carotenoids, serum beta-carotene, and retinol and risk of lung cancer in the alpha-tocopherol, beta-carotene cohort study. Am J Epidemiol. 2002 Sep 15;156(6):536-47.

Hollenberg NK. Flavanols and cardiovascular health: what is the evidence for chocolate and red wine? American Heart Association Scientific Sessions, Unofficial Satellite Symposium, November 11, 2001, Anaheim, California.

Hou DX. Potential mechanisms of cancer chemoprevention by anthocyanins. Curr Mol Med. 2003 Mar;3(2):149-59. Review.

Hou DX, Kai K, Li JJ, Lin S, Terahara N, Wakamatsu M, Fujii M, Young MR, Colburn N. Anthocyanidins inhibit activator protein 1 activity and cell transformation: structure-activity relationship and molecular mechanisms. Carcinogenesis. 2004 Jan;25(1):29-36. Epub September 26, 2003.

Howell AB. Cranberry proanthocyanidins and the maintenance of urinary tract health. Crit Rev Food Sci Nutr. 2002;42 Suppl 3:273-8. Review.

Howell AB, Foxman B. Cranberry juice and adhesion of antibiotic-resistant uropathogens. JAMA. 2002 Jun 19;287(23):3082-3. No abstract available.

Ito H, Kobayashi E, Takamatsu Y, Li SH, Hatano T, Sakagami H, Kusama K, Satoh K, Sugita D, Shimura S, Itoh Y, Yoshida T. Polyphenols from Eriobotrya japonica and their cytotoxicity against human oral tumor cell lines. Chem Pharm Bull (Tokyo). 2000 May;48(5):687-93.

Ito Y, Gajalakshmi KC, Sasaki R, Suzuki K, Shanta V. A study on serum carotenoid levels n breast cancer patients of Indian women in Chennai (Madras), India. J Epidemiol. 1999 Nov;9(5):306-14.

ang M, Pezzuto JM. Cancer chemopreventive activity of resveratrol. Drugs Exp Clin Res. 1999;25(2-3):65-77.

Kakegawa, et al. Inhibitory effects of tannins on hyaluronidase activation and on the degranulation from rat mesentery mast cells. Chem Pharm Bull. 1985; 33(11)3079-82.

Kaplan M, Hayek T, Raz A, Coleman R, Dornfeld L, Vaya J, Aviram M. Pomegranate juice supplementation to atherosclerotic mice reduces macrophage lipid peroxidation, cellular cholesterol accumulation and development of atherosclerosis. J Nutr. 2001 Aug;131(8):2082-9.

Keck AS, Finley JW. Cruciferous vegetables: cancer protective mechanisms of glucosinolate hydrolysis products and selenium. Integr Cancer Ther. 2004 Mar;3(1):5-12.

Kim ND, Mehta R, Yu W, Neeman I, Livney T, Amichay A, Poirier D, Nicholls P, Kirby A, Jiang W, Mansel R, Ramachandran C, Rabi T, Kaplan B, Lansky E. Chemopreventive and adjuvant therapeutic potential of pomegranate (Punica granatum) for human breast cancer. Breast Cancer Res Treat. 2002 Feb;71(3):203-17.

Kohlmeier L, Weterings KGC, Steck S, Kok FJ. Tea and cancer prevention: an evaluation of the epidemiologic literature. Nutr Cancer. 1997;27:1-13.

Kollar P, Hotolova H. [Biological effects of resveratrol and other constituents of wine.] Ceska Slov Farm. 2003 Nov;52(6):272-81. Review. Czech.

Krinsky NI. Micronutrients and their influence on mutagenicity and malignant transformation. Ann NY Acad Sci. 1993 May 28;686:229-42. Review.

Krinsky NI, Landrum JT, Bone RA. Biologic mechanisms of the protective role of lutein and zeaxanthin in the eye. Annu Rev Nutr. 2003;23:171-201. Epub February 27, 2003. Review.

Kris-Etherton PM, Keen CL. Evidence that the antioxidant flavonoids in tea and cocoa are beneficial for cardiovascular health. Curr Opin Lipidol. 2002 Feb;13(1):41-9. Review.

Kuttan R, et al. Collagen treated with (+) catechin becomes resistant to the action of mammalian collagenases. Experientia. 1981;37. Berhauser Verlag, Basel, Switzerland.

Lamson DW, Brignall MS. Antioxidants and cancer, part 3: quercetin. Altern Med Rev. 2000 Jun;5(3):196-208. Review.

LaVecchia C, Tavani A. Fruit and vegetables, and human cancer. Eur J Cancer Prev. 1998 Feb;7(1):3-8. Review.

Lee EH, Faulhaber D, Hanson KM, Ding W, Peters S, Kodali S, Granstein RD. Dietary lutein reduces ultraviolet radiation-induced inflammation and immunosuppression. J Invest Dermatol. 2004 Feb;122(2):510-7.

Lee IM, Cook NR, Manson JE, et al. Beta-carotene supplementation and incidence of cancer and cardiovascular disease: the Women's Health Study. J Natl Cancer Inst. 1999;91:2102-6.

Lee KW, Kim YJ, Kim DO, Lee HJ, Lee CY. Major phenolics in apple and their contribution to the total antioxidant capacity. J Agric Food Chem. 2003 Oct 22;51(22):6516-20.

Lee KW, Kim YJ, Lee HJ, Lee CY. Cocoa has more phenolic phytochemicals and a higher antioxidant capacity than teas and red wine. J Agric Food Chem. 2003 Dec 3;51(25):7292-5.

Li WG, Zhang XY, Wu YJ, Tian X. Anti-inflammatory effect and mechanism of proanthocyanidins from grape seeds. Acta Pharmacol Sin. 2001 Dec;22(12):1117-20.

Lopez-Velez M, Martinez-Martinez F, Del Valle-Ribes C. The study of phenolic compounds as natural antioxidants in wine. Crit Rev Food Sci Nutr. 2003;43(3):233-44. Review.

Lugasi A, Hovari J. Antioxidant properties of commercial alcoholic and nonalcoholic beverages. Nahrung. 2003 Apr;47(2):79-86.

Malik M, Zhao C, Schoene N, Guisti MM, Moyer MP, Magnuson BA. Anthocyanin-rich extract from Aronia meloncarpa E induces a cell cycle block in colon cancer but not normal colonic cells. Nutr Cancer. 2003;46(2):186-96.

Mazza G, Kay CD, Cottrell T, Holub BJ. Absorption of anthocyanins from blueberries and serum antioxidant status in human subjects. J Agric Food Chem. 2002 Dec 18;50(26):7731-7.

Mazza G, Miniati E. Small fruits. In: Anthocyanins in fruits, vegetables, and grains; Boca Raton, FL, CRC Press, 1993, 85-130.

McAlindon TE, Jacques P, Zhang Y, et al. Do antioxidant micronutrients protect against the development and progression of knee osteoarthritis? Arthritis Rheum. 1996;39:648-56.

McBride J. High-ORAC foods may slow aging. USDA Agricultural Research Service Web site. http://www.ars.usda.gov/is/pr/1999/990208.htm.

Micozzi MS, Beecher GR, Taylor PR, Khachik F. Carotenoid analyses of selected raw and cooked foods associated with a lower risk for cancer. J Natl Cancer Inst. 1990 Feb 21;82(4):282-5. Erratum in: J Natl Cancer Inst. 1990 Apr 18;82(8):715.

Milbury PE, Cao G, Prior RL, Blumberg J. Bioavailability of elderberry anthocyanins. Mech Ageing Dev. 2002 Apr 30;123(8):997-1006.

Miller MJ, Vergnolle N, McKnight W, Musah RA, Davison CA, Trentacosti AM, Thompson JH, Sandoval M, Wallace JL. Inhibition of neurogenic inflammation by the Amazonian herbal medicine sangre de grado. J Invest Dermatol. 2001 Sep;117(3):725-30.

Mittal A, Elmets CA, Katiyar SK. Dietary feeding of proanthocyanidins from grape seeds prevents photocarcinogenesis in SKH-1 hairless mice: relationship to decreased fat and lipid peroxidation. Carcinogenesis. 2003 Aug;24(8):1379-88. Epub June 5, 2003.

Moeller SM, Jacques PF, Blumberg JB. The potential role of dietary xanthophylls in cataract and age-related macular degeneration. J Am Coll Nutr. 2000 Oct;19 Suppl 5:522S-527S. Review.

Moyer RA, Hummer KE, Finn CE, Frei B, Wrolstad RE. Anthocyanins, phenolics, and anti-oxidant capacity in diverse small fruits: vaccinium, rubus, and ribes. J Agric Food Chem. 2002 Jan 30;50(3):519-25.

Murphy KJ, Chronopoulos AK, Singh I, Francis MA, Moriarty H, Pike MJ, Turner AH, Mann NJ, Sinclair AJ. Dietary flavanols and procyanidin oligomers from cocoa (Theobroma cacao) inhibit platelet function. Am J Clin Nutr. 2003 Jun;77(6):1466-73.

Nkondjock A, Ghadirian P. Intake of specific carotenoids and essential fatty acids and breast cancer risk in Montreal, Canada. Am J Clin Nutr. 2004 May;79(5):857-64.

O'Byrne DJ, Devaraj S, Grundy SM, Jialal I. Comparison of the antioxidant effects of Concord grape juice flavonoids alpha-tocopherol on markers of oxidative stress in healthy adults. Am J Clin Nutr. 2002 Dec;76(6):1367-74. [Co-sponsored by Welch's Foods Inc. (Concord, MA) and the National Institutes of Health.]

Omenn GS, Goodman GE, Thornquist MD, et al. Effects of a combination of beta carotene and vitamin A on lung cancer and cardiovascular disease. N Engl J Med. 1996;334:1150-5.

Orsini F, Pelizzoni F, Verotta L, Aburjai T, Rogers CB. Isolation, synthesis, and antiplatelet aggregation activity of resveratrol 3-O-beta-D-glucopyranoside and related compounds. J Nat Prod. 1997 Nov;60(11):1082-7.

Polyphenol flavonoid content and anti-oxidant activities of various juices: a comparative study. The Lipid Research Laboratory, Technion Faculty of Medicine, The Rappaport Family Institute for Research in the Medical Sciences and Rambam Medical Center, Haifa, Israel.

Robert AM, Tixier JM, Robert L, Legeais JM, Renard G. Effect of procyanidolic oligomers on the permeability of the blood-brain barrier. Pathol Biol (Paris). 2001 May;49(4):298-304.

Rock CL, Saxe GA, Ruffin MT 4th, et al. Carotenoids, vitamin A, and estrogen receptor status in breast cancer. Nutr Cancer. 1996;25:281-96.

Roy S, Khanna S, Alessio HM, Vider J, Bagchi D, Bagchi M, Sen CK. Anti-angiogenic property of edible berries. Free Radic Res. 2002 Sep;36(9):1023-31.

Schmidt K. Antioxidant vitamins and beta-carotene: effects on immunocompetence. Am J Clin Nutr. 1991 Jan;53 Suppl 1:383S-385S.

Schubert SY, Lansky EP, Neeman I. Antioxidant and eicosanoid enzyme inhibition properties of pomegranate seed oil and fermented juice flavonoids. J Ethnopharmacol. 1999 Jul;66(1):11-7.

Seddon JM, Ajani UA, Sperduto RD, et al. Dietary carotenoids, vitamins A, C, and E, and advanced age-related macular degeneration. Eye Disease Case-Control Study Group. JAMA. 1994;272:1413-20.

Seeram NP, Zhang Y, Nair MG. Inhibition of proliferation of human cancer cells and cyclooxygenase enzymes by anthocyanidins and catechins. Nutr Cancer. 2003;46(1):101-6.

Shapiro TA, Fahey JW, Wade KL, Stephenson KK, Talalay P. Chemoprotective glucosinolates and isothiocyanates of broccoli sprouts: metabolism and excretion in humans. Cancer Epidemiol Biomarkers Prev. 2001 May;10(5):501-8.

Shi J, Yu J, Pohorly JE, Kakuda Y. Polyphenolics in grape seeds—biochemistry and functionality. J Med Food. 2003 Winter;6(4):291-9.

Singletary KW, Meline B. Effect of grape seed proanthocyanidins on colon aberrant crypts and breast tumors in a rat dual-organ tumor model. Nutr Cancer. 2001;39(2):252-8.

Singletary KW, Stansbury MJ, Giusti M, Van Breemen RB, Wallig M, Rimando A. Inhibition of rat mammary tumorigenesis by Concord grape juice constituents. J Agric Food Chem. 2003 Dec 3;51(25):7280-6.

Slomski G. Lycopene. Gale encyclopedia of alternative medicine 2001.

Spencer JP, Schroeter H, Rechner AR, Rice-Evans C. Bioavailability of flavan-3-ols and procyanidins: gastrointestinal tract influences and their relevance to bioactive forms in vivo. Antioxid Redox Signal. 2001 Dec;3(6):1023-39. Review.

Steinmetz KA, Potter JD. Vegetables, fruit, and cancer prevention: a review. J Am Diet Assoc. 1996 Oct;96(10):1027-39. Review.

Stoclet JC, Kleschyov A, Andriambeloson E, Diebolt M, Andriantsitohaina R. Endothelial no release caused by red wine polyphenols. J Physiol Pharmacol. 1999 Dec;50(4):535-40.

Subarnas A, Wagner H. Analgesic and anti-inflammatory activity of the proanthocyanidin shellegueain A from Polypodium feei METT. Phytomedicine. 2000 Oct;7(5):401-5.

Tan WF, Lin LP, Li MH, Zhang YX, Tong YG, Xiao D, Ding J. Quercetin, a dietary-derived flavonoid, possesses antiangiogenic potential. Eur J Pharmacol. 2003 Jan 17;459(2-3):255-62.

Teikari JM, Rautalahti M, Haukka J, et al. Incidence of cataract operations in Finnish male smokers unaffected by alpha tocopherol or beta carotene supplements. J Epidemiol Community Health. 1998;52:468-72.

Tijburg LBM, Mattern T, Folts JD, Weisgerber UM, Katan MB. Tea flavonoids and cardiovascular diseases: a review. Crit Rev Food Sci Nutr. 1997;37:771-85.

Toniolo P, Van Kappel AL, Akhmedkhanov A, Ferrari P, Kato I, Shore RE, Riboli E. Serum carotenoids and breast cancer. Am J Epidemiol. 2001 Jun 15;153(12):1142-7.

Turujman SA, Wamer WG, Wei RR, Albert RH. Rapid liquid chromatographic method to distinguish wild salmon from aquacultured salmon fed synthetic astaxanthin. J AOAC Int. 1997 May-Jun;80(3):622-32.

van Doorn HE, van der Kruk GC, van Holst GJ. Large scale determination of glucosinolates in brussels sprouts samples after degradation of endogenous glucose. J Agric Food Chem. 1999 Mar;47(3):1029-34.

Vena JE, Graham S, Freudenheim J, et al. Diet in the epidemiology of bladder cancer in western New York. Nutr Cancer. 1992;18:255-64.

Vinson JA, Teufel K, Wu N. Red wine, de-alcoholised red wine, and especially grape juice, inhibit atherosclerosis in a hamster model. Atherosclerosis. 2001;156:1:67-72.

Vitale S, West S, Hallfrish J, et al. Plasma antioxidants and risk of cortical and nuclear cataract. Epidemiology. 1993;4:195-203.

Wang H, Cao G, Prior RL. Total antioxidant capacity of fruits. J Agr Food Chem. 1996;44(3):701-5.

Weisburger JH. Chemopreventive effects of cocoa polyphenols on chronic diseases. Exp Biol Med (Maywood). 2001 Nov;226(10):891-7. Review.

Yamagishi M, Natsume M, Osakabe N, Nakamura H, Furukawa F, Imazawa T, Nishikawa A, Hirose M. Effects of cacao liquor proanthocyanidins on PhIP-induced mutagenesis in vitro, and in vivo mammary and pancreatic tumorigenesis in female Sprague-Dawley rats. Cancer Lett. 2002 Nov 28;185(2):123-30.

Yamagishi M, Natsume M, Osakabe N, Okazaki K, Furukawa F, Imazawa T, Nishikawa A, Hirose M. Chemoprevention of lung carcinogenesis by cacao liquor proanthocyanidins in a male rat multi-organ carcinogenesis model. Cancer Lett. 2003 Feb 28;191(1):49-57.

Ye X, Krohn RL, Liu W, Joshi SS, Kuszynski CA, McGinn TR, Bagchi M, Preuss HG, Stohs SJ, Bagchi D. The cytotoxic effects of a novel IH636 grape seed proanthocyanidin extract on cultured human cancer cells. Mol Cell Biochem. 1999 Jun;196(1-2):99-108.

Zhang LX, et al. Carotenoids enhance hap junctional communication and inhibit lipid peroxidation in C3H/10T1/2 cells: relationship to their cancer chemopreventive action. Carcinogenesis. 1991;12:2109-14.

Zheng W, Sellers TA, Doyle TJ, et al. Retinol, antioxidant vitamins, and cancer of the upper digestive tract in a prospective cohort study of postmenopausal women. Am J Epidemiol. 1995;142:955-60.

Ziegler RG. Vegetables, fruits, and carotenoids and the risk of cancer. Am J Clin Nutr. 1991 Jan;53(Suppl1):251S-259S. Review.

Chapter 4

AAP 2000 red book: report of the committee on infectious diseases, 25th ed. American Academy of Pediatrics, 2000.

Afzal M, Al-Hadidi D, Menon M, Pesek J, Dhami MS. Ginger: an ethnomedical, chemical and pharmacological review. Drug Metabol Drug Interact. 2001;18(3-4):159-90. Review.

Agerholm-Larsen L, Raben A, Haulrik N, Hansen AS, Manders M, Astrup A. Effect of 8 week intake of probiotic milk products on risk factors for cardiovascular diseases. Eur J Clin Nutr. 2000 Apr; 54(4):288-97.

Aggarwal BB, Kumar A, Bharti AC. Anticancer potential of curcumin: preclinical and clinical studies. Anticancer Res. 2003 Jan-Feb;23(1A):363-98. Review.

Ahmed RS, Seth V, Banerjee BD. Influence of dietary ginger (Zingiber officinales Rosc) on antioxidant defense system in rat: comparison with ascorbic acid. Indian J Exp Biol. 2000 Jun;38(6):604-6.

Altman RD, Marcussen KC. Effects of a ginger extract on knee pain in patients with osteoarthritis. Arthritis Rheum. 2001;44:2531-8.

Anderson JW, Deakins DA, Floore TL, Smith BM, Whitis SE. Dietary fiber and coronary heart disease. Crit Rev Food Sci Nutr. 1990; 29:95-147.

Anderson JW, Gustafson NJ. Hypocholesterolemic effect of oat and bean products. Am J Clin Nutr. 1988;48:749-53.

Anderson JW, Gustafson NJ, Spencer DB, Tietyen J, Bryant CA. Serum lipid response of hypercholesterolemic men to single and divided doses of canned beans. Am J Clin Nutr. 1990; 51:1013-9.

Anderson JW, Johnstone BM, Cook-Newell ME. Meta-analysis of the effects of soy protein intake on serum lipids. N Engl J Med. 1995;333:276-82.

Antonio MA, Hawes SE, Hillier SL. The identification of vaginal Lactobacillus species and the demographic and microbiologic characteristics of women colonized by these species. J Infect Dis. 1999 Dec;180(6):1950-6.

Bazzano LA, He J, Ogden LG, Loria C, Vupputuri S, Myers L, Whelton PK. Legume consumption and risk of coronary heart disease in U.S. men and women. Arch Intern Med. 2001;161:2573-8.

Bengmark S. Colonic food: pre- and probiotics. Am J Gastroenterol. 2000 Jan;95Suppl 1:S5-S7. Review.

Bomba A, Nemcova R, Gancarcikova S, Herich R, Pistl J, Revajova V, Jonecova Z, Bugarsky A, Levkut M, Kastel R, Baran M, Lazar G, Hluchy M, Marsalkova S, Posivak J. The influence of omega-3 polyunsaturated fatty acids (omega-3 pufa) on lactobacilli adhesion to the intestinal mucosa and on immunity in gnotobiotic piglets. Berl Munch Tierarztl Wochenschr. 2003 Jul-Aug;116(7-8):312-6.

Borchers AT, Keen CL, Gershwin ME. The influence of yogurt/Lactobacillus on the innate and acquired immune response. Clin Rev Allergy Immunol. 2002 Jun;22(3):207-30. Review.

Bordia A, Verma SK, Srivastava KC. Effect of ginger (Zingiber officinale Rosc.) and fenugreek (Trigonella foenumgraecum L.) on blood lipids, blood sugar and platelet aggregation in patients with coronary artery disease. Prostaglandins Leukot Essent Fatty Acids. 1997;56:379-84.

Bressani R, Elías LG. The nutritional role of polyphenols in beans. In: Polyphenols in cereals and legumes. Hulse JH, ed. Ottawa, Canada, IDRC-145e, IDRC, 1979.

Bressani R, Elías LG, Braham JE. Reduction of digestibility of legume protein by tannins. In: Workshop on physiological effects of legumes in the laymen diet, XII International Congress of Nutrition, San Diego, California, August 1981.

Brouet I, Ohshima H. Curcumin, an anti-tumour promoter and anti-inflammatory agent, inhibits induction of nitric oxide synthase in activated macrophages. Biochem Biophys Res Commun. 1995 Jan 17;206(2):533-40.

Calabrese V, Scapagnini G, Colombrita C, Ravagna A, Pennisi G, Giuffrida Stella AM, Galli F, Butterfield DA. Redox regulation of heat shock protein expression in aging and neurodegenerative disorders associated with oxidative stress: a nutritional approach. Amino Acids. 2003 Dec;25(3-4):437-44. Epub November 7, 2003.

Caragay AB. Cancer-preventative foods and ingredients. Food Tech. 1992;46(4):65-8.

Carroll KK. Review of clinical studies on cholesterol lowering response to soy protein. J Am Diet Assoc. 1991;91:820-7.

Cav GH, Sofic E, Prior RL. Antioxidant capacity of tea and common vegetables. J Agr Food Chem. 1996 Nov;44(11):3426-31.

Cesarone MR, Belcaro G, Incandela L, Geroulakos G, Griffin M, Lennox A, DeSanctis MT, Acerbi G. Flight microangiopathy in medium-to-long distance flights: prevention of edema and microcirculation alterations with HR (Paroven, Venoruton; 0-(beta-hydroxyethyl)-rutosides): a prospective, randomized, controlled trial. J Cardiovasc Pharmacol Ther. 2002 Jan;7 Suppl 1:S17-S20.

Cesarone MR, Incandela L, DeSanctis MT, Belcaro G, Griffin M, Ippolito E, Acerbi G.

Treatment of edema and increased capillary filtration in venous hypertension with HR (Paroven, Venoruton; 0-(beta-hydroxyethyl)-rutosides): a clinical, prospective, placebo-controlled, randomized, dose-ranging trial. J Cardiovasc Pharmacol Ther. 2002 Jan;7 Suppl 1:S21-S24.

Chainani-Wu N. Safety and anti-inflammatory activity of curcumin: a component of turmeric (Curcuma longa). J Altern Complement Med. 2003 Feb;9(1):161-8. Review.

Chan MM. Inhibition of tumor necrosis factor by curcumin, a phytochemical. Biochem Pharmacol. 1995 May 26;49(11):1551-6.

Chan MM, Huang HI, Fenton MR, Fong D. In vivo inhibition of nitric oxide synthase gene expression by curcumin, a cancer preventive natural product with anti-inflammatory properties. Biochem Pharmacol. 1998 Jun 15;55(12):1955-62.

Chauhan DP. Chemotherapeutic potential of curcumin for colorectal cancer. Curr Pharm Des. 2002;8(19):1695-706. Review.

Chung WY, Yow CM, Benzie IF. Assessment of membrane protection by traditional Chinese medicine using a flow cytometric technique: preliminary findings. Redox Rep. 2003;8(1):31-3.

Conney AH, Lysz T, Ferraro T, Abidi TF, Manchand PS, Laskin JD, Huang MT. Inhibitory effect of curcumin and some related dietary compounds on tumor promotion and arachidonic acid metabolism in mouse skin. Adv Enzyme Regul. 1991;31:385-96. Review.

Cyong JA. A pharmacological study of the antiinflammatory activity of Chinese herbs— a review. Int J Acupuncture Electro-Ther Res. 1982;(7):173-202.

Danielsson G, Jungbeck C, Peterson K, Norgren L. A randomised controlled trial of micronised purified flavonoid fraction vs. placebo in patients with chronic venous disease. Eur J Vasc Endovasc Surg. 2002 Jan;23(1):73-6.

Delzenne N, Cherbut C, Neyrinck A. Prebiotics: actual and potential effects in inflammatory and malignant colonic diseases. Curr Opin Clin Nutr Metab Care. 2003 Sep;6(5):581-6. Review.

Deodhar SD, et al. Preliminary studies on anti-rheumatic activity of curcumin. Ind. J. Med. Res. 1980;71:632-4.

Dhuley JN. Anti-oxidant effects of cinnamon (Cinnamomum verum) bark and greater cardamom (Amomum subulatum) seeds in rats fed high fat diet. Indian J Exp Biol. 1999 Mar;37(3):238-42.

Dickerson C. Neuropeptide regulation of proinflammatory cytokine responses. J Leukoc Biol. 1998 May;63(5):602-5.

Dorai T, Cao YC, Dorai B, Buttyan R, Katz AE. Therapeutic potential of curcumin in human prostate cancer. III. Curcumin inhibits proliferation, induces apoptosis, and inhibits angiogenesis of LNCaP prostate cancer cells in vivo. Prostate. 2001 Jun 1;47(4):293-303.

D'Souza AL, et al. Probiotics in prevention of antibiotic associated diarrhoea: meta-analysis. Br Med J. 2002 Jun 8;324:1361.

Duenas M, Sun B, Hernandez T, Estrella I, Spranger MI. Proanthocyanidin composition in the seed coat of lentils (Lens culinaris L.). J Agric Food Chem. 2003 Dec

31;51(27):7999-8004.

Duvoix A, Morceau F, Delhalle S, Schmitz M, Schnekenburger M, Galteau MM, Dicato M, Diederich M. Induction of apoptosis by curcumin: mediation by glutathione S-transferase P1-1 inhibition. Biochem Pharmacol. 2003 Oct 15;66(8):1475-83.

Elmer GW. Probiotics: "living drugs." Am J Health Syst Pharm. 2001 Jun 15;58(12):1101-9. Review.

Fernandes G, Lawrence R, Sun D. Protective role of n-3 lipids and soy protein in osteoporosis. Prostaglandins Leukot Essent Fatty Acids. 2003 Jun;68(6):361-72. Review.

Fernandez-Orozco R, Zielinski H, Piskula MK. Contribution of low-molecular-weight antioxidants to the antioxidant capacity of raw and processed lentil seeds. Nahrung. 2003 Oct;47(5):291-9.

Floch MH, Hong-Curtiss J. Probiotics and functional foods in gastrointestinal disorders. Curr Gastroenterol Rep. 2001 Aug;3(4):343-50.

Food and Drug Administration HHS. Code of Federal Regulations. Office of the Federal Register National Archives and Records Administration. 1991. 21CFR, 131.200 (yogurt).

Friedrich MJ. A bit of culture for children: probiotics may improve health and fight disease. Jama. 2000 Sep 20;284(11):1365-6.

Fuhrman B, Rosenblat M, Hayek T, Coleman R, Aviram M. Ginger extract consumption reduces plasma cholesterol, inhibits LDL oxidation and attenuates development of atherosclerosis in atherosclerotic, apolipoprotein E-deficient mice. J Nutr. 2000 May;130(5):1124-31.

Gaon D, Garcia H, Winter L, Rodriguez N, Quintas R, Gonzalez SN, Oliver G. Effect of Lactobacillus strains and Saccharomyces boulardii on persistent diarrhea in children. Medicina (B Aires). 2003;63(4):293-8.

Gaon D, Garmendia C, Murrielo NO, de Cucco Games A, Cerchio A, Quintas R, Gonzalez SN, Oliver G. Effect of Lactobacillus strains (L. casei and L. acidophilus strains cerela) on bacterial overgrowth-related chronic diarrhea. Medicina (B Aires). 2002;62(2):159-63.

Geil PB, Anderson JW. Nutrition and health implications of dry beans: a review. J Am Coll Nutr. 1994 Dec;13(6):549-58. Review.

Ghosh S, Playford RJ. Bioactive natural compounds for the treatment of gastrointestinal disorders. Clin Sci (Lond). 2003 Jun;104(6):547-56. Review.

Grand RJ, et al. Lactose intolerance. UpToDate Electronic Database (Version 9.2). 2001.

Guardia T, Rotelli AE, Juarez AO, Pelzer LE. Anti-inflammatory properties of plant flavonoids. Effects of rutin, quercetin and hesperidin on adjuvant arthritis in rat. Farmaco. 2001 Sep;56(9):683-7.

Han SS, Keum YS, Chun KS, Surh YJ. Suppression of phorbol ester-induced NF-kappaB activation by capsaicin in cultured human promyelocytic leukemia cells. Arch Pharm Res. 2002 Aug;25(4):475-9.

Han SS, Keum YS, Seo HJ, Chun KS, Lee SS, Surh YJ. Capsaicin suppresses phorbol ester-induced activation of NF-kappaB/Rel and AP-1 transcription factors in mouse epidermis. Cancer Lett. 2001 Mar 26;164(2):119-26.

Ian SS, Keum YS, Seo HJ, Surh YJ. Curcumin suppresses activation of NF-kappaB and AP-1 induced by phorbol ester in cultured human promyelocytic leukemia cells. J Biochem Mol Biol. 2002 May 31;35(3):337-42.

Health and nutritional properties of probiotics in food including powder milk with live lactic acid bacteria—joint FAO/WHO expert consultation. Cordoba, Argentina, October 1-4, 2001 (EN). http://www.who.int/foodsafety/publications/fs_management/en/probiotics.pdf.

Herman C, Adlercreutz T, Goldin BR, et al. Soybean phytoestrogen intake and cancer risk. J Nutr 1995;125:757S-770S.

Ho C-T, Lee CY, Huang MT. Phenolic compounds in food and their effects on health I: analysis, occurrence, and chemistry. American Chemical Society Symposium Series 506, 315 pages, 1992. American Chemical Society, Washington, DC.

Ho C-T, Lee CY, Huang MT. Phenolic compounds in food and their effects on health II: antioxidants and cancer prevention. American Chemical Society Symposium Series 507, 402 pages, 1992. American Chemical Society, Washington, DC.

Hughes VL, Hillier SL. Microbiologic characteristics of Lactobacillus products used for colonization of the vagina. Obstet Gynecol. 1990;75:244-8.

Ihme N, Kiesewetter H, Jung F, Hoffmann KH, Birk A, Muller A, Grutzner KI. Leg oedema protection from a buckwheat herb tea in patients with chronic venous insufficiency: a single-centre, randomised, double-blind, placebo-controlled clinical trial. Eur J Clin Pharmacol. 1996;50(6):443-7.

Incandela L, Belcaro G, Renton S, DeSanctis MT, Cesarone MR, Bavera P, Ippolito E, Bucci M, Griffin M, Geroulakos G, Dugall M, Golden G, Acerbi G. HR (Paroven, Venoruton; 0-(beta-hydroxyethyl)-rutosides) in venous hypertensive microangiopathy: a prospective, placebo-controlled, randomized trial. J Cardiovasc Pharmacol Ther. 2002 Jan;7 Suppl 1:S7-S10.

Incandela L, Cesarone MR, DeSanctis MT, Belcaro G, Dugall M, Acerbi G. Treatment of diabetic microangiopathy and edema with HR (Paroven, Venoruton; 0-(beta-hydroxyethyl)-rutosides): a prospective, placebo-controlled, randomized study. J Cardiovasc Pharmacol Ther. 2002 Jan;7 Suppl 1:S11-S15.

Isolauri E. Probiotics: from anecdotes to clinical demonstration. J Allergy Clin Immunol. 2001 Dec;108(6):1062.

Ito K, Nakazato T, Yamato K, Miyakawa Y, Yamada T, Hozumi N, Segawa K, Ikeda Y, Kizaki M. Induction of apoptosis in leukemic cells by homovanillic acid derivative, capsaicin, through oxidative stress: implication of phosphorylation of p53 at Ser-15 residue by reactive oxygen species. Cancer Res. 2004 Feb 1;64(3):1071-8.

Jambunathan R, Singh U. Studies on desi and kabuli chickpea (Cicer arietinum l.) cultivars. 3. Mineral and trace element composition. J Agric Food Chem. 1981 Sep-Oct;29(5):1091-3.

Janssen PL, Meyboom S, van Staveren WA, et al. Consumption of ginger (Zingiber officinale Roscoe) does not affect ex vivo platelet thromboxane production in humans. Eur J Clin Nutr. 1996;50:772-4.

Jobin C, Bradham CA, Russo MP, Juma B, Narula AS, Brenner DA, Sartor RB. Curcumin blocks cytokine-mediated NF-kappa B activation and proinflammatory gene expression by inhibiting inhibitory factor I-kappa B kinase activity. J Immunol. 1999

Sep 15;163(6):3474–83.

Joe B, Lokesh BR. Effect of curcumin and capsaicin on arachidonic acid metabolism and lysosomal enzyme secretion by rat peritoneal macrophages. Lipids. 1997 Nov;32(11):1173–80.

Joe B, Lokesh BR. Role of capsaicin, curcumin and dietary n-3 fatty acids in lowering the generation of reactive oxygen species in rat peritoneal macrophages. Biochim Biophys Acta. 1994 Nov 10;1224(2):255–63.

Kan H, Onda M, Tanaka N, Furukawa K. [Effect of green tea polyphenol fraction on 1,2-dimethylhydrazine (DMH)-induced colorectal carcinogenesis in the rat.] Nippon Ika Daigaku Zasshi. 1996 Apr;63(2):106–16. Japanese.

Kang G, Kong PJ, Yuh YJ, Lim SY, Yim SV, Chun W, Kim SS. Curcumin suppresses lipopolysaccharide-induced cyclooxygenase-2 expression by inhibiting activator protein 1 and nuclear factor kappaB bindings in BV2 microglial cells. J Pharmacol Sci. 2004 Mar;94(3):325–8.

Kaur P, et al. Probiotics: potential pharmaceutical applications. Eur J Phar Sci. 2002 Feb;15:1–9.

Kawa JM, Taylor CG, Przybylski R. Buckwheat concentrate reduces serum glucose in streptozotocin-diabetic rats. J Agric Food Chem. 2003 Dec 3;51(25):7287–91.

Keating A, Chez RA. Ginger syrup as an antiemetic in early pregnancy. Altern Ther Health Med. 2002;8:89–91.

Kennedy AR. The evidence for soybean products as cancer preventive agents. J Nutr. 1995;125:733S–743S.

Kent HL. Epidemiology of vaginitis. Am J Obstet Gynecol 1991;165:1168–76.

Kiessling G, Schneider J, Jahreis G. Long-term consumption of fermented dairy products over 6 months increases HDL cholesterol. Eur J Clin Nutr. 2002 Sep;56(9):843–9.

Kihara N, de la Fuente SG, Fujino K, Takahashi T, Pappas TN, Mantyh CR. Vanilloid receptor-1 containing primary sensory neurones mediate dextran sulphate sodium induced colitis in rats. Gut. 2003 May;52(5):713–9.

Kikuzaki H, Nakatani N. Antioxidant effects of some ginger constituents. J Food Sci. 1993;58:1407.

Kiuchi F, et al. Inhibitors of prostaglandin biosynthesis from ginger. Chem Pharm Bull (Tokyo). 1982 Feb;30(2):754–7. Folia Pharmacologica Japonica. 1986 Oct;88(4):263–9.

Kolida S, Tuohy K, Gibson GR. Prebiotic effects of inulin and oligofructose. Br J Nutr. 2002 May;87 Suppl 2:S193–S197. Review.

Kurzer MS, Xu X. Dietary phytoestrogens. Ann Rev Nutr. 1997;17:353–81. Review.

Kwak JY. A capsaicin-receptor antagonist, capsazepine, reduces inflammation-induced hyperalgesic responses in the rat: evidence for an endogenous capsaicin-like substance. Neuroscience. 1998 Sep;86(2):619–26.

Lee YB, et al. Antioxidant property in ginger rhizome and its application to meat products. J Food Sci. 1986;51(1):20–3.

Li CH, Matsui T, Matsumoto K, Yamasaki R, Kawasaki T. Latent production of angiotensin I-converting enzyme inhibitors from buckwheat protein. J Pept Sci. 2002 Jun;8(6):267–74.

i SQ, Zhang QH. Advances in the development of functional foods from buckwheat. Crit Rev Food Sci Nutr. 2001 Sep;41(6):451-64. Review.

iacini A, Sylvester J, Li WQ, Huang W, Dehnade F, Ahmad M, Zafarullah M. Induction f matrix metalloproteinase-13 gene expression by TNF-alpha is mediated by MAP inases, AP-1, and NF-kappaB transcription factors in articular chondrocytes. Exp Cell Res. 2003 Aug 1;288(1):208-17.

ien HC, Sun WM, Chen YH, et al. Effects of ginger on motion sickness and gastric low-wave dysrhythmias induced by circular vection. Am J Physiol Gastrointest Liver Physiol. 2003;284:G481-G489.

iepke C, Adermann K, Raida M, Magert HJ, Forssmann WG, Zucht HD. Human milk provides peptides highly stimulating the growth of bifidobacteria. Eur J Biochem. 2002 Jan;269(2):712-8.

im GP, Chu T, Yang F, Beech W, Frautschy SA, Cole GM. The curry spice curcumin reduces oxidative damage and amyloid pathology in an Alzheimer transgenic mouse. J Neurosci. 2001 Nov 1;21(21):8370-7.

iu N, Huo G, Zhang L, Zhang X. [Effect of Zingiber officinale Rosc on lipid peroxidation in hyperlipidemia rats.] Wei Sheng Yan Jiu. 2003 Jan;32(1):22-3. Chinese.

u P, Lai BS, Liang P, Chen ZT, Shun SQ. [Antioxidation activity and protective effection of ginger oil on DNA damage in vitro.] Zhongguo Zhong Yao Za Zhi. 2003 Sep;28(9):873-5. Chinese.

umb AB. Effect of dried ginger on human platelet function. Thromb Haemost. 1994;71:110-1.

Majamaa H, Isolauri E. Probiotics: a novel approach in the management of food allergy. Allergy Clin Immunol. 1997 Feb;99(2):179-85.

Menne E, Guggenbuhl N, Roberfroid M. Fn-type chicory inulin hydrolysate has a prebiotic effect in humans. J Nutr. 2000 May;130(5):1197-9.

Messina M, Messina V. Increasing use of soy foods and their potential role in cancer prevention. J Am Diet Assoc. 1991;91:836-40.

Messina M, Messina V. The simple soybean and your health. New York, Avery Publishing Company, 1994.

Messina MJ, Persky V, Setchell KD, et al. Soy intake and cancer risk: a review of the in vitro and in vivo data. Nutr Cancer. 1994;21(2):113-31.

Metchnikoff E. The prolongation of life: optimistic studies. New York, G.P. Putnam's Sons, 1908.

Miraglia del Giudice M Jr, De Luca MG, Capristo C. Probiotics and atopic dermatitis. A new strategy in atopic dermatitis. Dig Liver Dis. 2002 Sep;34 Suppl 2:S68-S71.

Mitchell JA. Role of nitric oxide in the dilator actions of capsaicin-sensitive nerves in the rabbit coronary circulation. Neuropeptides. 1997 Aug;31(4):333-8.

Murosaki S, Muroyama K, Yamamoto Y, Yoshikai Y. Antitumor effect of heat-killed Lactobacillus plantarum L-137 through restoration of impaired interleukin-12 production in tumor-bearing mice. Cancer Immunol Immunother. 2000 Jun;49(3):157-64.

Nestel P, Cehun M, Pomeroy S, Abbey M, Duo L, Weldon G. Cholesterol-lowering effects of sterol esters and non-esterified sitostanol in margarine, butter and low-fat foods. Eur J Cardio Nurs. 2001;55:1084-90.

Nyirjesy P, et al. Over-the-counter and alternative medicines in the treatment of chronic vaginal symptoms. Obstet Gynecol. 1997;90:50-3.

Oh GS, Pae HO, Seo WG, Kim NY, Pyun KH, Kim IK, Shin M, Chung HT. Capsazepine, a vanilloid receptor antagonist, inhibits the expression of inducible nitric oxide synthase gene in lipopolysaccharide-stimulated RAW264.7 macrophages through the inactivation of nuclear transcription factor-kappa B. Int Immunopharmacol. 2001 Apr;1(4):777-84.

Ohta T, Nakatsugi S, Watanabe K, Kawamori T, Ishikawa F, Morotomi M, Sugie S, Toda T, Sugimura T, Wakabayashi K. Inhibitory effects of Bifidobacterium-fermented soy milk on 2-amino-1-methyl-6-phenylimidazo[4,5-b]pyridine-induced rat mammary carcinogenesis, with a partial contribution of its component isoflavones. Carcinogenesis. 2000 May;21(5):937-41.

Onoda M, Inano H. Effect of curcumin on the production of nitric oxide by cultured rat mammary gland. Nitric Oxide. 2000 Oct;4(5):505-15.

Ostrakhovitch EA, Afanas'ev IB. Oxidative stress in rheumatoid arthritis leukocytes: suppression by rutin and other antioxidants and chelators. Biochem Pharmacol. 2001 Sep 15;62(6):743-6.

Pan MH, Lin-Shiau SY, Lin JK. Comparative studies on the suppression of nitric oxide synthase by curcumin and its hydrogenated metabolites through down-regulation of IkappaB kinase and NFkappaB activation in macrophages. Biochem Pharmacol. 2000 Dec 1;60(11):1665-76.

Park JM, Adam RM, Peters CA, Guthrie PD, Sun Z, Klagsbrun M, Freeman MR. AP-1 mediates stretch-induced expression of HB-EGF in bladder smooth muscle cells. Am J Physiol. 1999 Aug;277(2 Pt 1):C294-C301.

Patel PS, Varney ML, Dave BJ, Singh RK. Regulation of constitutive and induced NF-kappaB activation in malignant melanoma cells by capsaicin modulates interleukin-8 production and cell proliferation. J Interferon Cytokine Res. 2002 Apr;22(4):427-35.

Peterson KF, Dufour S, Befroy D, Garcia R, Shulman GI. Impaired activity in the insulin-resistant offspring of patients with type 2 diabetes. N Engl J Med. 2004 Feb 12;350:664-71.

Petruzzellis V, Troccoli T, Candiani C, Guarisco R, Lospalluti M, Belcaro G, Dugall M. Oxerutins (Venoruton): efficacy in chronic venous insufficiency—a double-blind, randomized, controlled study. Angiology. 2002 May-Jun;53(3):257-63.

Phan TT, See P, Lee ST, Chan SY. Protective effects of curcumin against oxidative damage on skin cells in vitro: its implication for wound healing. J Trauma. 2001 Nov;51(5):927-31.

Plummer SM, Holloway KA, Manson MM, Munks RJ, Kaptein A, Farrow S, Howells L. Inhibition of cyclo-oxygenase 2 expression in colon cells by the chemopreventive agent curcumin involves inhibition of NF-kappaB activation via the NIK/IKK signalling complex. Oncogene. 1999 Oct 28;18(44):6013-20.

Pongrojpaw D, Chiamchanya C. The efficacy of ginger in prevention of post-operative nausea and vomiting after outpatient gynecological laparoscopy. J Med Assoc Thai. 2003;86:244-50.

Potter SM. Overview of proposed mechanisms for the hypocholesterolemic effect of soy. J Nutr. 1995;125:606S-611S.

Potter SM, Bakhit RM, Essex-Sorlie DL, et al. Depression of plasma cholesterol in men by consumption of baked products containing soy protein. Am J Clin Nutr. 1993;58:501-6.

Prasad NS, Raghavendra R, Lokesh BR, Naidu KA. Spice phenolics inhibit human PMNL 5-lipoxygenase. Prostaglandins Leukot Essent Fatty Acids. 2004 Jun;70(6):521-8.

Rafter JJ. Scientific basis of biomarkers and benefits of functional foods for reduction of disease risk: cancer. Br J Nutr. 2002 Nov;88 Suppl 2:S219-S224. Review.

Ramirez-Tortosa MC, Mesa MD, Aguilera MC, Quiles JL, Baro L, Ramirez-Tortosa CL, Martinez-Victoria E, Gil A. Oral administration of a turmeric extract inhibits LDL oxidation and has hypocholesterolemic effects in rabbits with experimental atherosclerosis. Atherosclerosis. 1999 Dec;147(2):371-8.

Rao BN. Bioactive phytochemicals in Indian foods and their potential in health promotion and disease prevention. Asia Pac J Clin Nutr. 2003;12(1):9-22. Review.

Rao CV, et al. Antioxidant activity of curcumin and related compounds. Lipid peroxide formation in experimental inflammation. Cancer Res 1993;55:259.

Rautava S, Isolauri E. The development of gut immune responses and gut microbiota: effects of probiotics in prevention and treatment of allergic disease. Curr Issues Intest Microbiol. 2002 Mar;3(1):15-22.

Reid G, Bocking A. The potential for probiotics to prevent bacterial vaginosis and preterm labor. Am J Obstet Gynecol. 2003 Oct;189(4):1202-8. Review.

Reid G, Howard J, Gan BS. Can bacterial interference prevent infection? Trends Microbiol. 2001 Sep;9(9):424-8.

Reuter G. [Probiotics—possibilities and limitations of their application in food, animal feed, and in pharmaceutical preparations for men and animals.] Berl Munch Tierarztl Wochenschr. 2001 Nov-Dec;114(11-12):410-9. Review. German.

Rolfe RD. The role of probiotic cultures in the control of gastrointestinal health. J Nutr. 2000 Feb;130 (Suppl 2S):396S-402S. Review.

Roos K, et al. Effect of recolonization with "interfering" streptococci on recurrences of acute and secretory otitis media in children: randomized placebo controlled trial. Br Med J. 2001;32:210.

Saavedra JM, Tschernia A. Human studies with probiotics and prebiotics: clinical implications. Br J Nutr. 2002 May;87 Suppl 2:S241-S246. Review.

Saito Y. The antioxidant effects of petroleum ether soluble and insoluble fractions from spices. Eiyo To Shokuryo. 1976;29:505-10.

Satoskar RR, Shah SJ, Shenoy SG. Evaluation of anti-inflammatory property of curcumin (diferuloyl methane) in patients with postoperative inflammation. Int J Clin Pharmacol Ther Toxicol. 1986 Dec;24(12):651-4.

Schiffrin EJ, Blum S. Interactions between the microbiota and the intestinal mucosa. Eur J Clin Nutr. 2002 Aug;56 Suppl 3:S60-S64. Review.

Schultz M, Scholmerich J, Rath HC. Rationale for probiotic and antibiotic treatment strategies in inflammatory bowel diseases. Dig Dis. 2003;21(2):105-28. Review.

Setchell KD, Lydeking-Olsen E. Dietary phytoestrogens and their effect on bone: evidence from in vitro and in vivo, human observational, and dietary intervention studies. Am J Clin Nutr. 2003 Sep;78 (Suppl 3):593S-609S. Review.

Shah BH, Nawaz Z, Pertani SA, Roomi A, Mahmood H, Saeed SA, Gilani AH. Inhibitory effect of curcumin, a food spice from turmeric, on platelet-activating factor- and arachidonic acid-mediated platelet aggregation through inhibition of thromboxane formation and Ca2+ signaling. Biochem Pharmacol. 1999 Oct 1;58(7):1167-72.

Shalev E, Battino S, Weiner E, Colodner R, Keness Y. Ingestion of yogurt containing Lactobacillus acidophilus compared with pasteurized yogurt as prophylaxis for recurrent candidal vaginitis and bacterial vaginosis. Arch Fam Med. 1996 Nov-Dec;5(10):593-6.

Sharma SC, et al. Lipid peroxide formation in experimental inflammation. Biochem Pharmacol. 1972;21:1210.

Shutler SM, Bircher GM, Tredger JA, Morgan LM, Walker AF, Low AG. The effect of daily baked bean (Phaseolus vulgaris) consumption on the plasma lipid levels of young, normo-cholesterolaemic men. Br J Nutr. 1989;61:257-65.

Simpson HCR, Lousley S, Geekie M, Simpson RW, Carter RD, Hockaday TDR, Mann JI. A high carbohydrate leguminous fibre diet improves all aspects of diabetic control. Lancet. 1981;i:1-5.

Singh S, Aggarwal BB. Activation of transcription factor NF-kappa B is suppressed by curcumin (diferuloylmethane) [corrected]. J Biol Chem. 1995 Oct 20;270(42):24995-5000. Erratum in: J Biol Chem. 1995 Dec 15;270(50):30235.

Singh S, Natarajan K, Aggarwal BB. Capsaicin (8-methyl-N-vanillyl-6-nonenamide) is a potent inhibitor of nuclear transcription factor-kappa B activation by diverse agents. J Immunol. 1996 Nov 15;157(10):4412-20.

Smith BM, Whitis SE. Dietary fiber and coronary heart disease. Crit Rev Food Sci Nutr. 1990;29:95-147.

Sobel JD. Overview of vaginitis. UpToDate Electronic Database (Version 9.2), 2001.

Soliman KF, Mazzio EA. In vitro attenuation of nitric oxide production in C6 astrocyte cell culture by various dietary compounds. Proc Soc Exp Biol Med. 1998 Sep;218(4):390-7.

Soni KB, Kuttan R. Effect of oral curcumin administration on serum peroxides and cholesterol levels in human volunteers. Ind J Physiol Pharmacol. 1992;(36):273, 293.

Sreekanth KS, Sabu MC, Varghese L, Manesh C, Kuttan G, Kuttan R. Antioxidant activity of Smoke Shield in-vitro and in-vivo. J Pharm Pharmacol. 2003 Jun;55(6):847-53.

Srimal R, Dhawan B. Pharmacology of diferuloyl methane (curcumin), a non-steroidal anti-inflammatory agent. J Pharm Pharmac. 1973;(25):447-52.

Srinivas L, et al. Turmerin: a water-soluble antioxidant peptide from turmeric. Arch Biochem Biophy. 1992;(292):617.

Srivasta R, Srimal RC. Modification of certain inflammation-induced biochemical changes by curcumin. Indian J Med Res. 1985;(81):215-23.

Srivastava KC. Effect of onion and ginger consumption on platelet thromboxane pro-uction in humans. Prostaglandins Leukot Essent Fatty Acids. 1989;35:183-5.

rivastava KC. Effects of aqueous extracts of onion, garlic and ginger on platelet aggregation and metabolism of arachidonic acid in the blood vascular system: in vitro study. Prostaglandins Leukot Med. 1984;13:227-35.

rivastava KC. Isolation and effects of some ginger components on platelet aggregation and eicosanoid biosynthesis. Prostaglandins Leukot Med. 1986;25:187-98.

rivastava KC, Mustafa T. Ginger (Zingiber officinale) and rheumatic disorders. Med Hypotheses. 1989 May;29(1):25-8.

rivastava KC, Mustafa T. Ginger (Zingiber officinale) in rheumatic and musculoskeletal disorders. Med Hypotheses. 1992 Dec;39(4):342-8.

tavric B. Antimutagens and anticarcinogens in foods. Food Chem Toxicol. 1994 Jan;32(1):79-90. Review.

teele MG. The effect on serum cholesterol levels of substituting milk with a soya beverage. Aust J Nutr Diet. 1992;49:24-8.

uekawa M, et al. [Pharmacological studies on ginger. IV. Effect of (6)-shogaol on the arachidonic cascade.] Nippon Yakurigaku Zasshi. 1986 Oct;88(4):263-9.

urh YJ. Anti-tumor promoting potential of selected spice ingredients with antioxidative and anti-inflammatory activities: a short review. Food Chem Toxicol. 2002 Aug;40(8):1091-7. Review.

urh YJ, Chun KS, Cha HH, Han SS, Keum YS, Park KK, Lee SS. Molecular mechanisms underlying chemopreventive activities of anti-inflammatory phytochemicals: down-regulation of COX-2 and iNOS through suppression of NF-kappa B activation. Mutat Res. 2001 Sep 1;480-1, 243-68. Review.

urh YJ, Han SS, Keum YS, Seo HJ, Lee SS. Inhibitory effects of curcumin and capsaicin on phorbol ester-induced activation of eukaryotic transcription factors, NF-kappaB and AP-1. Biofactors. 2000;12(1-4):107-12.

usan M, Rao MNA. Induction of glutathione S-transferase activity by curcumin in mice. Arznheim Foresh. 1992;42:962.

Tannock GW. Normal microflora. New York, Chapman and Hall, 1995.

Tjendraputra E, Tran VH, Liu-Brennan D, Roufogalis BD, Duke CC. Effect of ginger constituents and synthetic analogues on cyclooxygenase-2 enzyme in intact cells. Bioorg Chem. 2001 Jun;29(3):156-63.

Turmeric for treating health ailments. Invented by Van Bich Nguyen, College Park, MD. No assignee. U.S. Patent 6,048,533. Issued April 11, 2000. This patent (and U.S. Patent 5,897,865, issued April 27, 1999) covers the therapeutic use of the common spice curmeric (Curcuma longa) for the treatment of skin disorders such as acne, blemishes, psoriasis, dandruff, dry skin, discoloration, irritation, and sun damage.

Udani J. Lactobacillus acidophilus to prevent traveler's diarrhea. Altern Med Alert. 1999;2:53-5.

Vanderhoof JA. Probiotics: future directions. Am J Clin Nutr. 2001 Jun;73:1152S-1155S.

Van Kessel K, Assefi N, Marrazzo J, Eckert L. Common complementary and alternative therapies for yeast vaginitis and bacterial vaginosis: a systematic review. Obstet Gynecol Surv. 2003 May;58(5):351-8. Review.

Wang CC, Chen LG, Lee LT, Yang LL. Effects of 6-gingerol, an antioxidant from ginger, on inducing apoptosis in human leukemic HL-60 cells. In Vivo. 2003 Nov-Dec;17(6):641–5.

Weisburger JH. Tea and health: the underlying mechanisms. Proc Soc Exp Biol Med. 1999 Apr;220(4):271–5. Review.

Wood JR, et al. In vitro adherence of Lactobacillus species to vaginal epithelial cells. Am J Obstet Gynecol. 1985;153:740–3.

Zeneb MB, et al. Dairy (yogurt) augments fat loss and reduces central adiposity during energy restriction in obese subjects. FASEB. 2003;17(5):A1088.

Zhang J, Nagasaki M, Tanaka Y, Morikawa S. Capsaicin inhibits growth of adult T-cell leukemia cells. Leuk Res. 2003 Mar;27(3):275–83.

Chapter 5

Abbey M, Noakes M, Belling GB, Nestel PJ. Partial replacement of saturated fatty acids with almonds or walnuts lowers total plasma cholesterol and low-density-lipoprotein cholesterol. Am J Clin Nutr. 1994 May;59(5):995–9.

Abila B, Richens A, Davies JA. Anticonvulsant effects of extracts of the West African black pepper, Piper guineense. J Ethnopharmacol. 1993 Jun;39(2):113–7.

Ahn SC, Oh WK, Kim BY, Kang DO, Kim MS, Heo GY, Ahn JS. Inhibitory effects of rosmarinic acid on Lck SH2 domain binding to a synthetic phosphopeptide. Planta Med. 2003 Jul;69(7):642–6.

Ahsan H, Parveen N, Khan NU, Hadi SM. Pro-oxidant, antioxidant and cleavage activities on DNA of curcumin and its derivatives demethoxycurcumin and bisdemethoxycurcumin. Chem Biol Interact. 1999 Jul 1;121(2):161–75.

Akgul A, Kivanc M. Inhibitory effects of selected Turkish spices and oregano components on some foodborne fungi. Int J Food Microbiol. 1988 May;6(3):263–8.

Akoachere JF, Ndip RN, Chenwi EB, et al. Antibacterial effect of Zingiber officinale and Garcinia kola on respiratory tract pathogens. East Afr Med J. 2002 Nov;79(11):588–92.

Ali BH, Blunden G. Pharmacological and toxicological properties of Nigella sativa. Phytother Res. 2003 Apr;17(4):299–305. Review.

al-Sereiti MR, Abu-Amer KM, Sen P. Pharmacology of rosemary (Rosmarinus officinalis Linn.) and its therapeutic potentials. Indian J Exp Biol. 1999 Feb;37(2):124–30. Review.

Anderson RA, Broadhurst CL, Polansky MM, Schmidt WF, Khan A, Flanagan VP, Schoene NW, Graves DJ. Isolation and characterization of polyphenol type-A polymers from cinnamon with insulin-like biological activity. Diabetes Res Clin Pract. 2003 Dec;62(3):139–48.

Anuradha CV, Ravikumar P. Restoration on tissue antioxidants by fenugreek seeds (Trigonella foenum graecum) in alloxan-diabetic rats. Indian J Physiol Pharmacol. 2001 Oct;45(4):408–20.

Ao P, Hu S, Zhao A. Institute of Chinese Material Medica, China Academy of Traditional Chinese Medicine, Beijing 100700. [Essential oil analysis and trace element study the roots of Piper nigrum L.] Zhongguo Zhong Yao Za Zhi. 1998 Jan;23(1):42-3, . Chinese.

biser JL, Klauber N, Rohan R, et al. Curcumin is an in vivo inhibitor of angiogen-s. Mol Med. 1998 Jun;4(6):376-83.

eias F, Valentao P, Andrade PB, Ferreres F, Seabra RM. Flavonoids and phenolic acids sage: influence of some agricultural factors. J Agric Food Chem. 2000 ec;48(12):6081-4.

sai A, Nakagawa K, Miyazawa T. Antioxidative effects of turmeric, rosemary and cap-:um extracts on membrane phospholipid peroxidation and liver lipid metabolism in ice. Biosci Biotechnol Biochem. 1999 Dec;63(12):2118-22.

igamboula CF, Uyttendaele and M, Debevere J. Antimicrobial effect of spices and erbs on Shigella sonnei and Shigella flexneri. J Food Prot. 2003 Apr;66(4):668-73.

igamboula CF, Uyttendaele and M, Debevere J. Inhibitory effect of thyme and basil sential oils, carvacrol, thymol, estragol, linalool and p-cymene towards Shigella sonnei d S. flexneri. Food Microbio. 2004 Feb;21(1):33-42.

allal RS, Jacobsen DW, Robinson K. Homocysteine: update on a new risk factor. Cleve lin J Med. 1997 Nov-Dec 31;64(10):543-9.

ierhaus A, Zhang Y, Quehenberger P, Luther T, Haase M, Muller M, Mackman N, iegler R, Nawroth PP. The dietary pigment curcumin reduces endothelial tissue factor ne expression by inhibiting binding of AP-1 to the DNA and activation of NF-kappa . Thromb Haemost. 1997 Apr;77(4):772-82.

ode A. Ginger is an effective inhibitor of HCT116 human colorectal carcinoma in vo. Paper presented at the Frontiers in Cancer Prevention Research Conference, hoenix, Arizona, October 26-30, 2003.

roadhurst CL, Polansky MM, Anderson RA. Insulin-like biological activity of culinary id medicinal plant aqueous extracts in vitro. J Agric Food Chem. 2000 Mar;48(3):849-2.

alucci L, Pinzino C, Zandomeneghi M, et al. Effects of gamma-irradiation on the free idical and antioxidant contents in nine aromatic herbs and spices. J Agric Food Chem. 003 Feb 12; 51(4):927-34.

hithra V, Leelamma S. Coriandrum sativum changes the levels of lipid peroxides and :tivity of antioxidant enzymes in experimental animals. Indian J Biochem Biophys. 999 Feb;36(1):59-61.

hithra V, Leelamma S. Hypolipidemic effect of coriander seeds (Coriandrum sativum): iechanism of action. Plant Foods Hum Nutr. 1997;51(2):167-72.

ipriani B, Borsellino G, Knowles H, Tramonti D, Cavaliere F, Bernardi G, Battistini L, rosnan CF. Curcumin inhibits activation of Vgamma9Vdelta2 T cells by phosphoanti-ens and induces apoptosis involving apoptosis-inducing factor and large scale DNA agmentation. J Immunol. 2001 Sep 15;167(6):3454-62.

osentino S, Tuberoso CI, Pisano B, Satta M, Mascia V, Arzedi E, Palmas F. In-vitro ntimicrobial activity and chemical composition of Sardinian Thymus essential oils. Lett ppl Microbiol. 1999 Aug;29(2):130-5.

)apkevicius A, van Beek TA, Lelyveld GP, van Veldhuizen A, de Groot A, Linssen JP, Ven-kutonis R. Isolation and structure elucidation of radical scavengers from Thymus vulgaris leaves. J Nat Prod. 2002 Jun;65(6):892-6.

Delaquis PJ, Stanich K, Girard B. et al. Antimicrobial activity of individual and mixe fractions of dill, cilantro, coriander and eucalyptus essential oils. Int J Food Microbio 2002 Mar 25;74(1-2):101-9.

Deshpande UR, Gadre SG, Raste AS, et al. Protective effect of turmeric (Curcum longa L.) extract on carbon tetrachloride-induced liver damage in rats. Indian J Ex Biol. 1998 Jun;36(6):573-7.

Devasena T, Menon VP. Enhancement of circulatory antioxidants by fenugreek durin 1,2-dimethylhydrazine-induced rat colon carcinogenesis. J Biochem Mol Biol Biophys 2002 Aug;6(4):289-92.

Dorai T, Cao YC, Dorai B, et al. Therapeutic potential of curcumin in human prostat cancer. III. Curcumin inhibits proliferation, induces apoptosis, and inhibits angiogenes of LNCaP prostate cancer cells in vivo. Prostate. 2001 Jun 1;47(4):293-303.

Dorman HJ, Deans SG. Antimicrobial agents from plants: antibacterial activity of plan volatile oils. J Appl Microbiol. 2000 Feb;88(2):308-16.

Dragland S, Senoo H, Wake K, Holte K, Blomhoff R. Several culinary and medicin₂ herbs are important sources of dietary antioxidants. J Nutr. 2003 May;133(5):1286-90

Elgayyar M, Draughon FA, Golden DA, Mount JR. Antimicrobial activity of essentia oils from plants against selected pathogenic and saprophytic microorganisms. J Foo Prot. 2001 Jul;64(7):1019-24.

Exarchou V, Nenadis N, Tsimidou M, Gerothanassis IP, Troganis A, Boskou D. Antioxi dant activities and phenolic composition of extracts from Greek oregano, Greek sage and summer savory. J Agric Food Chem. 2002 Sep 11;50(19):5294-9.

Ficker CE, Arnason JT, Vindas PS, et al. Inhibition of human pathogenic fungi by ethno botanically selected plant extracts. Mycoses. 2003 Feb;46(1-2):29-37.

Fischer-Rasmussen W, Kjaer SK, Dahl C, et al. Ginger treatment of hyperemesis gravi darum. Eur J Obstet Gynecol Reprod Biol. 1990;38:19-24.

Gagandeep, Dhanalakshmi S, Mendiz E, Rao AR, Kale RK. Chemopreventive effects o Cuminum cyminum in chemically induced forestomach and uterine cervix tumors ir murine model systems. Nutr Cancer. 2003;47(2):171-80.

Genet S, Kale RK, Baquer NZ. Alterations in antioxidant enzymes and oxidative damage in experimental diabetic rat tissues: effect of vanadate and fenugreek (Trigonel lafoenum graecum). Mol Cell Biochem. 2002 Jul;236(1-2):7-12.

Gray AM, Flatt PR. Insulin-releasing and insulin-like activity of the traditional anti-dia betic plant Coriandrum sativum (coriander). Br J Nutr. 1999 Mar;81(3):203-9.

Gururaj A, Kelakavadi M, Venkatesh D, et al. Molecular mechanisms of anti-angiogenic effect of curcumin. Biochem Biophys Res Commun. 2002 Oct 4;297(4):934.

Haddad JJ. Redox regulation of pro-inflammatory cytokines and IkappaB-alpha/NF-kappaB nuclear translocation and activation. Biochem Biophys Res Commun. 2002 Aug 30;296(4):847-56. Erratum in: Biochem Biophys Res Commun. 2003 Feb 7;301(2):625.

Hammer KA, Carson CF, Riley TV. Antimicrobial activity of essential oils and other plant extracts. J Appl Microbiol. 1999 Jun;86(6):985-90.

...raguchi H, Saito T, Ishikawa H, Date H, Kataoka S, Tamura Y, Mizutani K. Antiper-
idative components in Thymus vulgaris. Planta Med. 1996 Jun;62(3):217-21.

...raguchi H, Saito T, Okamura N, Yagi A. Inhibition of lipid peroxidation and super-
ide generation by diterpenoids from Rosmarinus officinalis. Planta Med. 1995
...g;61(4):333-6.

...daka H, Ishiko T, Furunashi T, et al. Curcumin inhibits interleukin 8 production and
...hances interleukin 8 receptor expression on the cell surface: impact on human pan-
...eatic carcinoma cell growth by autocrine regulation. Cancer. 2002 Sep 15;96(6):1206-

...tokoto H, Morozumi S, Wauke T, Sakai S, Kurata H. Inhibitory effects of spices on
...owth and toxin production of toxigenic fungi. Appl Environ Microbiol. 1980
...or;39(4):818-22.

...oughton P. Sage, alternative treatment to Alzheimer's drug. Research presented at the
...itish Pharmaceutical Conference in Harrogate, September 15-17, 2003.

...uang CD, Tliba O, Panettieri RA Jr, Amrani Y. Bradykinin induces interleukin-6 pro-
...uction in human airway smooth muscle cells: modulation by Th2 cytokines and dex-
...nethasone. Am J Respir Cell Mol Biol. 2003 Mar;28(3):330-8.

...npari-Radosevich J, Deas S, Polansky MM, et al. Regulation of PTP-1 and insulin
...ceptor kinase by fractions from cinnamon: implications for cinnamon regulation of
...sulin signaling. Horm Res. 1998 Sep;50(3):177-82.

...poushi K, Azuma K, Ito H, Horie H, Higashio H. [6]-Gingerol inhibits nitric oxide
...nthesis in activated J774.1 mouse macrophages and prevents peroxynitrite-induced
...xidation and nitration reactions. Life Sci. 2003 Nov 14;73(26):3427-37.

...getia GC, Baliga MS, Venkatesh P, Ulloor JN. Influence of ginger rhizome (Zingiber
...ficinale Rosc) on survival, glutathione and lipid peroxidation in mice after whole-
...ody exposure to gamma radiation. Radiat Res. 2003 Nov;160(5):584-92.

...alemba D, Kunicka A. Antibacterial and antifungal properties of essential oils. Curr
...led Chem. 2003 May;10(10):813-29. Review.

...ang BY, Chung SW, Chung W, et al. Inhibition of interleukin-12 production in
...opolysaccharide-activated macrophage by curcumin. Eur J Pharmacol. 1999
...ov;384(2-3):191-5.

...ang BY, Song YJ, Kim KM, et al. Curcumin inhibits Th1 cytokine profile in CD4+ T
...ells by suppressing interleukin-12 production in macrophages. Br J Pharmacol. 1999
...ep;128(2):380-4.

...aur C, Kapoor CH. antioxidant activity and total phenolic content of some Asian veg-
...ables. Int J Food Sci Tech. 2002 Feb;37(2):153.

...elm MA, Nair MG, Strasburg GM, DeWitt DL. Antioxidant and cyclooxygenase
...hibitory phenolic compounds from Ocimum sanctum Linn. Phytomedicine. 2000
...lar;7(1):7-13.

...han A, Safdar M, Ali Khan MM, Khattak KN, Anderson RA. Cinnamon improves glu-
...ose and lipids of people with type 2 diabetes. Diabetes Care. 2003 Dec;26(12):3215-8.

...han N, Sharma S, Sultana S. Nigella sativa (black cumin) ameliorates potassium bro-
...late-induced early events of carcinogenesis: diminution of oxidative stress. Hum Exp

Toxicol. 2003 Apr;22(4):193-203.

Kikuzaki H, Kawai Y, Nakatani N. 1,1-Diphenyl-2-picrylhydrazyl radical-scavengin active compounds from greater cardamom (Amomum subulatum Roxb.). J Nutr Sc Vitaminol (Tokyo). 2001 Apr;47(2):167-71.

Kim DO, Lee KW, Lee HJ, Lee CY. Vitamin C equivalent antioxidant capacit (VCEAC) of phenolic phytochemicals. J Agric Food Chem. 2002 Jun 19;50(13):3713 7.

Kiuchi F, et al. Inhibition of prostaglandin and leukotriene biosynthesis by gingerols an diarylheptanoids. Chem Pharm Bull. 1992;40:387-91.

Kulevanova S, Kaftandzieva A, Dimitrovska A, et al. Investigation of antimicrobia activity of essential oils of several Macedonian Thymus L. species (Lamiaceae). Bo Chim Farm. 2000 Nov-Dec 31;139(6):276-80.

Lagouri V, Boskou D. Nutrient antioxidants in oregano. Int J Food Sci Nutr. 199 Nov;47(6):493-7.

Lambert RJ, Skandamis PN, Coote PJ, Nychas GJ. A study of the minimum inhibitor concentration and mode of action of oregano essential oil, thymol and carvacrol. J App Microbiol. 2001 Sep;91(3):453-62.

Langmead L, Dawson C, Hawkins C, Banna N, Loo S, Rampton DS. Antioxidant effect of herbal therapies used by patients with inflammatory bowel disease: an in vitro study Aliment Pharmacol Ther. 2002 Feb;16(2):197-205.

Li D, Zimmerman TL, Thevananther S, Lee HY, Kurie JM, Karpen SJ. Interleukin- beta-mediated suppression of RXR:RAR transactivation of the Ntcp promoter is JNK dependent. J Biol Chem. 2002 Aug 30;277(35):31416-22. Epub June 24, 2002.

Lim GP, Chu T, Yang F, et al. The curry spice curcumin reduces oxidative damage an amyloid pathology in an Alzheimer transgenic mouse. J Neurosci. 2001 Nov 1;21(21):8370-7.

Madar Z, Stark AH. New legume sources as therapeutic agents. Br J Nutr. 2002 Dec;8 Suppl 3:S287-S292. Review.

Malencic D, Gasic O, Popovic M, Boza P. Screening for antioxidant properties of Salvi reflexa hornem. Phytother Res. 2000 Nov;14(7):546-8.

Martinez-Tome M, Jimenez AM, Ruggieri S, et al. Antioxidant properties of Mediter- ranean spices compared with common food additives. J Food Prot. 200 Sep;64(9):1412-9.

Matsingou TC, Petrakis N, Kapsokefalou M, Salifoglou A. Antioxidant activity o organic extracts from aqueous infusions of sage. J Agric Food Chem. 2003 Nov 5;51(23):6696-701.

Meeker HG, Linke HA. The antibacterial action of eugenol, thyme oil, and relate essential oils used in dentistry. Compendium 1988 Jan;9(1):32, 34-5, 38 passim.

Mujumdar AM, Dhuley JN, Deshmukh VK, et al. Anti-inflammatory activity o piperine. Jpn J Med Sci Biol. 1990 Jun;43(3):95-100.

Murcia MA, Egea I, Romojaro F, Parras P, Jimenez AM, Martinez-Tome M. Antioxidan evaluation in dessert spices compared with common food additives. Influence of irradi- ation procedure. J Agric Food Chem. 2004 Apr 7;52(7):1872-81.

Nair S, Nagar R, Gupta R. Antioxidant phenolics and flavonoids in common Indian foods. J Assoc Physicians India. 1998 Aug;46(8):708-10.

Nakamura K, Yasunaga Y, Segawa T, et al. Curcumin down-regulates AR gene expression and activation in prostate cancer cell lines. Int J Oncol. 2002 Oct;21(4):825-30.

Natarajan C, Bright JJ. Peroxisome proliferator-activated receptor-gamma agonists inhibit experimental allergic encephalomyelitis by blocking IL-2 production, IL-12 signaling and Th1 differentiation. Genes Immun. 2002 Apr;3(2):59-70.

Nature Immunology Online. 2001;10.1038/ni732.

Olszewska M, Glowacki R, Wolbis M, Bald E. Quantitative determination of flavonoids in the flowers and leaves of Prunus spinosa L. Acta Pol Pharm. 2001 May-Jun 30;58(3):199-203.

Opalchenova G, Obreshkova D. Comparative studies on the activity of basil—an essential oil from Ocimum basilicum L.—against multidrug resistant clinical isolates of the genera Staphylococcus, Enterococcus and Pseudomonas by usi. J Microbiol Methods. Jul;54(1):105-10.

Orafidiya LO, Oyedele AO, Shittu AO, Elujoba AA. The formulation of an effective topical antibacterial product containing Ocimum gratissimum leaf essential oil. Int J Pharm. 2001 Aug 14;224(1-2):177-83.

Otsuka H, Fujioka S, Komiya T, et al. [Studies on anti-inflammatory agents. VI. Anti-inflammatory constituents of Cinnamomum sieboldii Meissn (author's transl)]. Yakugaku Zasshi. 1982 Jan;102(2):162-72.

Ouattara B, Simard RE, Holley RA, et al. Antibacterial activity of selected fatty acids and essential oils against six meat spoilage organisms. Int J Food Microbiol. 1997 Jul 22;37(2-3):155-62.

Pandian RS, Anuradha CV, Viswanathan P. Gastroprotective effect of fenugreek seeds (Trigonella foenum graecum) on experimental gastric ulcer in rats. J Ethnopharmacol. 2002 Aug;81(3):393-7.

Park SY, Kim DS. Discovery of natural products from Curcuma longa that protect cells from beta-amyloid insult: a drug discovery effort against Alzheimer's disease. J Nat Prod. 2002 Sep;65(9):1227-31.

Perry EK, Pickering AT, Wang WW, Houghton PJ, Perry NS. Medicinal plants and Alzheimer's disease: from ethnobotany to phytotherapy. J Pharm Pharmacol. 1999 May;51(5):527-34.

Perry EK, Pickering AT, Wang WW, Houghton P, Perry NS. Medicinal plants and Alzheimer's disease: integrating ethnobotanical and contemporary scientific evidence. J Altern Complement Med. 1998 Winter;4(4):419-28. Review.

Perry NS, Houghton PJ, Sampson J, Theobald AE, Hart S, Lis-Balchin M, Hoult JR, Evans P, Jenner P, Milligan S, Perry EK. In-vitro activity of S. lavandulaefolia (Spanish sage) relevant to treatment of Alzheimer's disease. J Pharm Pharmacol. 2001 Oct;53(10):1347-56.

Perry NS, Houghton PJ, Theobald A, Jenner P, Perry EK. In-vitro inhibition of human erythrocyte acetylcholinesterase by Salvia lavandulaefolia essential oil and constituent terpenes. J Pharm Pharmacol. 2000 Jul;52(7):895-902. Erratum in: J Pharm Pharmacol. 2000 Dec;52(12):203.

Qin B, Nagasaki M, Ren M, Bajotto G, Oshida Y, Sato Y. Cinnamon extract prevents the insulin resistance induced by a high-fructose diet. Horm Metab Res. 2004 Feb;36(2):119-25.

Qin B, Nagasaki M, Ren M, Bajotto G, Oshida Y, Sato Y. Cinnamon extract (traditional herb) potentiates in vivo insulin-regulated glucose utilization via enhancing insulin signaling in rats. Diabetes Res Clin Pract. 2003 Dec;62(3):139-48.

Quale JM, Landman D, Zaman MM, et al. In vitro activity of Cinnamomum zeylanicum against azole resistant and sensitive Candida species and a pilot study of cinnamon for oral candidiasis. Am J Chin Med. 1996;24(2):103-9.

Rasooli I, Mirmostafa SA. Bacterial susceptibility to and chemical composition of essential oils from Thymus kotschyanus and Thymus persicus. J Agric Food Chem. 2003 Apr 9;51(8):2200-5.

Salh B, Assi K, Templeman V, Parhar K, Owen D, Gomez-Munoz A, Jacobson K. Curcumin attenuates DNB-induced murine colitis. Am J Physiol Gastrointest Liver Physiol. 2003 Jul;285(1):G235-43. Epub March 13, 2003.

Shah BH, Nawaz Z, Pertani SA, et al. Inhibitory effect of curcumin, a food spice from turmeric, on platelet-activating factor- and arachidonic acid-mediated platelet aggregation through inhibition of thromboxane formation and Ca2+ signa. Biochem Pharmacol. 1999 Oct 1;58(7):1167-72.

Shoba G, Joy D, Joseph T, Majeed M, Rajendran R, Srinivas PS. Influence of piperine on the pharmacokinetics of curcumin in animals and human volunteers. Planta Med. 1998 May;64(4):353-6.

Singh A, Singh SP, Bamezai R. Modulatory potential of clocimum oil on mouse skin papillomagenesis and the xenobiotic detoxication system. Food Chem Toxicol. 1999 Jun;37(6):663-70.

Singh G, Kapoor IP, Pandey SK, et al. Studies on essential oils: part 10; antibacterial activity of volatile oils of some spices. Phytother Res. 2002 Nov;16(7):680-2.

Srivastava KC, Mustafa T. Ginger (Zingiber officinale) and rheumatic disorders. Med Hypothesis. 1989;29:25-8.

Srivastava KC, Mustafa T. Ginger (Zingiber officinale) in rheumatism and musculoskeletal disorders. Med Hypothesis. 1992;39:342-8.

Sunila ES, Kuttan G. Immunomodulatory and antitumor activity of Piper longum Linn. and piperine. J Ethnopharmacol. 2004 Feb;90(2-3):339-46.

Tabak M, Armon R, Potasman I, Neeman I. In vitro inhibition of Heliobacter pylori by extracts of thyme. J Appl Bacteriol. 1996 Jun;80(6):667-72.

Takacsova M, Pribela A, Faktorova M. Study of the antioxidative effects of thyme, sage, juniper and oregano. Nahrung. 1995;39(3):241-3.

Takenaga M, Hirai A, Terano T, et al. In vitro effect of cinnamic aldehyde, a main component of Cinnamomi cortex, on human platelet aggregation and arachidonic acid metabolism. J Pharmacobiodyn. 1987 May;10(5):201-8.

Thirunavukkarasu V, Anuradha CV, Viswanathan P. Protective effect of fenugreek (Trigonella foenum graecum) seeds in experimental ethanol toxicity. Phytother Res. 2003 Aug;17(7):737-43.

Tildesley NT, Kennedy DO, Perry EK, Ballard CG, Savelev S, Wesnes KA, Scholey AB. Salvia lavandulaefolia (Spanish sage) enhances memory in healthy young volunteers. Pharmacol Biochem Behav. 2003 Jun;75(3):669-74.

Uma Devi P. Radioprotective, anticarcinogenic and antioxidant properties of the Indian holy basil, Ocimum sanctum (Tulasi). Indian J Exp Biol. 2001 Mar;39(3):185-90.

Valenzuela A, Sanhueza J, Nieto S. Cholesterol oxidation: health hazard and the role of antioxidants in prevention. Biol Res. 2003;36(3-4):291-302. Review.

Valero M, Salmeron MC. Antibacterial activity of 11 essential oils against Bacillus cereus in tyndallized carrot broth. Int J Food Microbiol. Aug 15;85(1-2):73-81.

VanderEnde DS, Morrow JD. Release of markedly increased quantities of prostaglandin D2 from the skin in vivo in humans after the application of cinnamic aldehyde. J Am Acad Dermatol. 2001 Jul;45(1):62-7.

Vrinda B, Uma Devi P. Radiation protection of human lymphocyte chromosomes in vitro by orientin and vicenin. Mutat Res. 2001 Nov 15;498(1-2):39-46.

Wigler I, Grotto I, Caspi D, Yaron M. The effects of Zintona EC (a ginger extract) on symptomatic gonarthritis. Osteoarthritis Cartilage. 2003 Nov;11(11):783-9.

Wills RB, Scriven FM, Greenfield H. Nutrient composition of stone fruit (Prunus spp.) cultivars: apricot, cherry, nectarine, peach and plum. J Sci Food Agric. 1983 Dec;34(12):1383-9.

Wuthi-udomler M, Grisanapan W, Luanratana O, Caichompoo W. Antifungal activity of Curcuma longa grown in Thailand. Southeast Asian J Trop Med Public Health. 2000;31 Suppl 1:178-82.

Youdim KA, Deans SG. Beneficial effects of thyme oil on age-related changes in the phospholipid C20 and C22 polyunsaturated fatty acid composition of various rat tissues. Biochem Biophys Acta. 1999 Apr 19;1438(1):140-6.

Youdim KA, Deans SG. Dietary supplementation of thyme (Thymus vulgaris L.) essential oil during the lifetime of the rat: its effects on the antioxidant status in liver, kidney and heart tissues. Mech Ageing Dev. 1999 Sep 8;109(3):163-75.

Youdim KA, Deans SG. On the antioxidant status and fatty acid composition of the ageing rat brain. Br J Nutr. 2000 Jan;83(1):87-93.

Zeng HH, Tu PF, Zhou K, Wang H, Wang BH, Lu JF. Antioxidant properties of phenolic diterpenes from Rosmarinus officinalis. Acta Pharmacol Sin. 2001 Dec;22(12):1094-8.

Zheng GQ, Kenney PM, Lam LK. Anethofuran, carvone, and limonene: potential cancer chemopreventive agents from dill weed oil and caraway oil. Planta Med. 1992 Aug; 58(4):338-41.

Zheng W, Wang SY. Antioxidant activity and phenolic compounds in selected herbs. J Agric Food Chem. 2001 Nov;49(11):5165-70.

Zoladz P, Raudenbush B, Lilley S. Cinnamon perks performance. Paper presented at the annual meeting of the Association for Chemoreception Sciences, held in Sarasota, Florida, April 21-25, 2004.

Chapter 6

Beal MF. Aging, energy, and oxidative stress in neurodegenerative diseases. Ann Neurol.

1995;38:357–66.

Beal MF. Does impairment of energy metabolism result in excitotoxic neuronal death in neurodegenerative diseases? Ann Neurol. 1992;31:119–23.

Blass JP, Gibson GE, Shimada M, Kihara T, Watanabe M, Kurinioto K. Brain carbohydrate metabolism and dementia. In: Biochemistry of dementia, Burman D, Pennock CA, eds. London, Wiley, 1980, 121–34.

Blass JP, Sheu K-FR, Cederbaum JM. Energy metabolism in disorders of the nervous system. Rev Neurol (Paris). 1988;144:543–63.

Blass JP, Sheu, K-FR, Tanzi R. a-Ketoglutarate dehydrogenase in Alzheimer's disease. In: Energy metabolism in neurodegenerative diseases, Fiskum G, ed. New York, Plenum, 1996, 185–92.

Borchers AT, Keen CL, Gershwin ME. Mushrooms, tumors, and immunity: an update. Exp Biol Med (Maywood). 2004 May;229(5):393–406. Review.

Davis PK, Johnson GV. Monoclonal antibody Alz-50 reacts with bovine and human ser albumin. J Neurosci Res. 1994;39(5):589–94.

Fabrizi C, Businaro R, Lauro GM, Starace G, Fumagalli L. Activated alpha2macroglobulin increase beta-amyloid (25-35)-induced toxicity in LA-N5 human neuroblastoma cells. Exp Neurol. 1999;155(2):252–9.

Huu Toan N, Ngan Tam L. The efficacy of alpha-PSP on coronary heart disease in the staff of Cho Ray Hospital with HDL-cholesterol and lipidemia disorders: an open-label, non-comparative study. Cho Ray Hospital, 201B-Nguyen Chi Thanh Street, 5th district. Ho Chi Minh City, Vietnam, 2001.

Kidd PM. The use of mushroom glucans and proteoglycans in cancer treatment. Altern Med Rev. 2000 Feb;5(1):4–27. Review.

Manohar V, Talpur NA, Echard BW, Lieberman S, Preuss HG. Effects of a water-soluble extract of maitake mushroom on circulating glucose/insulin concentrations in KK mice. Diabetes Obes Metab. 2002 Jan;4(1):43–8.

Mattson MP. Mechanism of neuronal degeneration and preventive approaches: Quickening the pace of AD research. Neurobiol Aging. 1994;15 Suppl 2:S121–S125.

Mayell M. Maitake extracts and their therapeutic potential. Altern Med Rev. 2001 Feb;6(1):48–60. Review.

Mesco ER, Timiras PS. Tau-ubiquitin protein conjugates Ia human cell Hine. Mech Ageing Dev. 1991;61(l):1–9.

Preuss U, Mandelhow EM. Mitotic phosphorylation of tau protein in neuronal cell lines resembles phosphorylation in Alzheimer's disease. Eur J Cell Biol. 1998;76(3):176–84.

Sawatsri S, Yankunthong W. Neurofood may prevent neuron vulnerability in human neuroblastoma cells. (Preliminary Data)

Talpur N, Echard B, Dadgar A, Aggarwal S, Zhuang C, Bagchi D, Preuss HG. Effects of maitake mushroom fractions on blood pressure of Zucker fatty rats. Res Commun Mol Pathol Pharmacol. 2002;112(1-4):68–82.

Talpur NA, Echard BW, Fan AY, Jaffari O, Bagchi D, Preuss HG. Antihypertensive and metabolic effects of whole maitake mushroom powder and its fractions in two rat strains. Mol Cell Biochem. 2002 Aug;237(1-2):129-36.

Talpur N, Echard BW, Yasmin T, Bagchi D, Preuss HG. Effects of niacin-bound chromium, maitake mushroom fraction SX and (-)-hydroxycitric acid on the metabolic syndrome in aged diabetic Zucker fatty rats. Mol Cell Biochem. 2003 Oct;252(1-2):369-77.

Tasawat N, Tayraukham S. A study on alpha-PSP towards a better quality of life as a part of symptomatic changes in 767 Asian diabetic patients. Macro Food Tech Co. Ltd., 2002.

Wasser SP. Medicinal mushrooms as a source of antitumor and immunomodulating polysaccharides. Appl Microbiol Biotechnol. 2002 Nov;60(3):258-74. Epub September 10, 2002. Review.

Chapter 7

Alabovskii VV, Boldyrev AA, Vinokurov AA, Gallant S, Chesnokov DN. Comparison of protective effects of carnosine and acetylcarnosine during cardioplegia. Biull Eksp Biol Med. 1999 Mar;127(3):290-4.

Andrews M, Gallagher-Allred C. The role of zinc in wound healing. Adv Wound Care. 1999 Apr;12(3):137-8. Review.

Ayello EA, Thomas DR, Litchford MA. Nutritional aspects of wound healing. Home Health Nurse. 1999 Nov-Dec;17(11):719-29, quiz 730. Review.

Bakardjiev A, Bauer K. Biosynthesis, release, and uptake of carnosine in primary cultures. Biochemistry (Mosc). 2000 Jul;65(7):779-82.

Belury MA. Inhibition of carcinogenesis by conjugated linoleic acid: potential mechanisms of action. J Nutr. 2002 Oct;132(10):2995-8. Review.

Belury MA, Mahon A, Banni S. The conjugated linoleic acid (CLA) isomer, t10c12-CLA, is inversely associated with changes in body weight and serum leptin in subjects with type 2 diabetes mellitus. J Nutr. 2003 Jan;133(1):257S-260S. Review.

Beyer RE. An analysis of the role of coenzyme Q in free radical generation and as an anti-oxidant. Biochem Cell Biol. 1992 Jun;70(6):390-403. Review.

Bierhaus A, Chevion S, Chevion M, Hofmann M, Quehenberger P, Illmer T, Luther T, Berentshtein E, Tritschler H, Muller M, Wahl P, Ziegler R, Nawroth PP. Advanced glycation end product-induced activation of NF-kappaB is suppressed by alpha-lipoic acid in cultured endothelial cells. Diabetes. 1997 Sep;46(9):1481-90.

Cakatay U, Telci A, Kayali R, Sivas A, Akcay T. Effect of alpha-lipoic acid supplementation on oxidative protein damage in the streptozotocin-diabetic rat. Res Exp Med (Berl). 2000 Feb;199(4):243-51.

Crane FL. Biochemical functions of coenzyme Q10. J Am Coll Nutr. 2001 Dec;20(6):591-8. Review.

Cuzzocrea S, Thiemermann C, Salvemini D. Potential therapeutic effect of antioxidant therapy in shock and inflammation. Curr Med Chem. 2004 May;11(9):1147-62.

Dadmarz M, vd Burg C, Milakofsky L, Hofford JM, Vogel WH. Effects of stress on amino acids and related compounds in various tissues of fasted rats. Life Sci. 1998;63(16):1485-91.

Decker EA, Livisay SA, Zhou S. A re-evaluation of the antioxidant activity of purified carnosine. Biochemistry (Mosc). 2000 Jul;65(7):766-70.

Deev LI, Goncharenko EN, Baizhumanov AA, Akhalaia MIa, Antonova SV, Shestakova SV. Protective effect of carnosine in hyperthermia. Biull Eksp Biol Med. 1997 Jul;124(7):50-2.

Dollwet HH, Sorenson JR. Roles of copper in bone maintenance and healing. Biol Trace Elem Res. 1988 Dec;18:39-48. Review.

El-seweidy MM, El-Swefy SE, Ameen RS, Hashem RM. Effect of age receptor blocker and/or anti-inflammatory coadministration in relation to glycation, oxidative stress and cytokine production in stz diabetic rats. Pharmacol Res. 2002 May;45(5):391-8.

Evans JL, Goldfine ID. Alpha-lipoic acid: a multifunctional antioxidant that improves insulin sensitivity in patients with type 2 diabetes. Diabetes Technol Ther. 2000 Autumn;2(3):401-13. Review.

Fuchs J, Milbradt R. Antioxidant inhibition of skin inflammation induced by reactive oxidants: evaluation of the redox couple dihydrolipoate/lipoate. Skin Pharmacol. 1994;7(5):278-84.

Gaullier JM, Halse J, Høye K, Kristiansen K, Fagertun H, Vik H, Gudmundsen O. Conjugated linoleic acid supplementation for 1 y reduces body fat mass in healthy overweight humans. Am J Clin Nutr. 2004;79(6):1118-25.

Gutierrez A, Anderstam B, Alvestrand A. Amino acid concentration in the interstitium of human skeletal muscle: a microdialysis study. Eur J Clin Invest. 1999 Nov;29(11):947-52.

Hagen TM, Liu J, Lykkesfeldt J, Wehr CM, Ingersoll RT, Vinarsky V, Bartholomew JC, Ames BN. Feeding acetyl-L-carnitine and lipoic acid to old rats significantly improves metabolic function while decreasing oxidative stress. Proc Natl Acad Sci USA. 2002 Feb 19;99(4):1870-5. Erratum in: Proc Natl Acad Sci USA. 2002 May 14;99(10):7184.

Hammes HP, Du X, Edelstein D, Taguchi T, Matsumura T, Ju Q, Lin J, Bierhaus A, Nawroth P, Hannak D, Neumaier M, Bergfeld R, Giardino I, Brownlee M. Benfotiamine blocks three major pathways of hyperglycemic damage and prevents experimental diabetic retinopathy. Nat Med. 2003 Mar;9(3):294-9. Epub February 18, 2003.

Han D, Handelman G, Marcocci L, Sen CK, Roy S, Kobuchi H, Tritschler HJ, Flohe L, Packer L. Lipoic acid increases de novo synthesis of cellular glutathione by improving cystine utilization. Biofactors. 1997;6(3):321-38.

Hannappel E, Huff T. The thymosins. Prothymosin alpha, parathymosin, and beta-thymosins: structure and function. Vitam Horm. 2003;66:257-96. Review.

Hipkiss AR, Preston JE, Himsworth DT, Worthington VC, Keown M, Michaelis J, Lawrence J, Mateen A, Allende L, Eagles PA, Abbott NJ. Pluripotent protective effects of carnosine, a naturally occurring dipeptide. Ann NY Acad Sci. 1998 Nov 20;854:37-

53.

Hoppel C. The role of carnitine in normal and altered fatty acid metabolism. Am J Kidney Dis. 2003 Apr;41(4 Suppl 4):S4-S12. Review.

Houseknecht KL, Vanden Heuvel JP, Moya-Camarena SY, Portocarrero CP, Peck LW, Nickel KP, Belury MA. Dietary conjugated linoleic acid normalizes impaired glucose tolerance in the Zucker diabetic fatty fa/fa rat. Biochem Biophys Res Commun. 1998 Mar 27;244(3):678-82. Erratum in: Biochem Biophys Res Commun. 1998 Jun 29;247(3):911.

Huff T, Muller CS, Otto AM, Netzker R, Hannappel E. Beta-thymosins, small acidic peptides with multiple functions. Int J Biochem Cell Biol. 2001 Mar;33(3):205-20. Review.

Ikeda S, Toyoshima K, Yamashita K. Dietary sesame seeds elevate alpha- and gamma-tocotrienol concentrations in skin and adipose tissue of rats fed the tocotrienol-rich fraction extracted from palm oil. J Nutr. 2001 Nov;131(11):2892-7.

Kagan VE, Shvedova A, Serbinova E, Khan S, Swanson C, Powell R, Packer L. Dihydrolipoic acid—a universal antioxidant both in the membrane and in the aqueous phase. Reduction of peroxyl, ascorbyl and chromanoxyl radicals. Biochem Pharmacol. 1992 Oct 20;44(8):1637-49.

Kamal-Eldin A, Appelqvist LA. The chemistry and antioxidant properties of tocopherols and tocotrienols. Lipids. 1996 Jul;31(7):671-701. Review.

Kocak G, Aktan F, Canbolat O, Ozogul C, Elbeg S, Yildizoglu-Ari N, Karasu C. Alpha-lipoic acid treatment ameliorates metabolic parameters, blood pressure, vascular reactivity and morphology of vessels already damaged by streptozotocin-diabetes. Diabetes Nutr Metab. 2000 Dec;13(6):308-18.

Komarcevic A. [The modern approach to wound treatment.] Med Pregl. 2000 Jul-Aug;53(7-8):363-8. Review. Croatian.

Kunt T, et al. Alpha-lipoic acid reduces expression of vascular cell adhesion molecule-1 and endothelial adhesion of human monocytes after stimulation with advanced glycation end products. Clin Sci (Lond). 1999 Jan;96(1):75-82.

Lee JW, Miyawaki H, Bobst EV, Hester JD, Ashraf M, Bobst AM. Improved functional recovery of ischemic rat hearts due to singlet oxygen scavengers histidine and carnosine. J Mol Cell Cardiol. 1999 Jan;31(1):113-21.

Linetsky M, James HL, Ortwerth BJ. Spontaneous generation of superoxide anion by human lens proteins and by calf lens proteins ascorbylated in vitro. Exp Eye Res. 1999 Aug;69(2):239-48.

Malinda KM, Sidhu GS, Mani H, Banaudha K, Maheshwari RK, Goldstein AL, Kleinman HK. Thymosin beta4 accelerates wound healing. J Invest Dermatol. 1999 Sep;113(3):364-8.

Melhem MF, Craven PA, Derubertis FR. Effects of dietary supplementation of alpha-lipoic acid on early glomerular injury in diabetes mellitus. J Am Soc Nephrol. 2001 Jan;12(1):124-33.

Melhem MF, Craven PA, Liachenko J, DeRubertis FR. Alpha-lipoic acid attenuates hyperglycemia and prevents glomerular mesangial matrix expansion in diabetes. J Am Soc Nephrol. 2002 Jan;13(1):108-16.

Meyer M, Pahl HL, Baeuerle PA. Regulation of the transcription factors NF-kappa B and AP-1 by redox changes. Chem Biol Interact. 1994 Jun;91(2-3):91-100.

Meyer M, Schreck R, Baeuerle PA. H2O2 and antioxidants have opposite effects on activation of NF-kappa B and AP-1 in intact cells: AP-1 as secondary antioxidant-responsive factor. EMBO J. 1993 May;12(5):2005-15.

Midaoui AE, Elimadi A, Wu L, Haddad PS, de Champlain J. Lipoic acid prevents hypertension, hyperglycemia, and the increase in heart mitochondrial superoxide production. Am J Hypertens. 2003 Mar;16(3):173-9.

Mzhel'skaia TI, Boldyrev AA. The biological role of carnosine in excitable tissues. Zh Obshch Biol. 1998 May-Jun;59(3):263-78.

Nachbar F, Korting HC. The role of vitamin E in normal and damaged skin. J Mol Med. 1995 Jan;73(1):7-17. Review.

Naguib Y, Hari SP, Passwater R Jr, Huang D. Antioxidant activities of natural vitamin E formulations. J Nutr Sci Vitaminol (Tokyo). 2003 Aug;49(4):217-20.

Obrenovich ME, Monnier VM. Vitamin B1 blocks damage caused by hyperglycemia. Sci Aging Knowledge Environ. 2003 Mar 12;2003(10):PE6.

Ookawara T, Kawamura N, Kitagawa Y, Taniguchi N. Site-specific and random fragmentation of Cu,Zn-superoxide dismutase by glycation reaction. Implication of reactive oxygen species. J Biol Chem. 1992 Sep 15;267(26):18505-10.

Packer L, Kraemer K, Rimbach G. Molecular aspects of lipoic acid in the prevention of diabetes complications. Nutrition. 2001 Oct;17(10):888-95. Review.

Packer L, Roy S, Sen CK. A-lipoic acid: a metabolic antioxidant and potential redox modulator of transcription. Adv Pharmacol. 1996;38:79-101.

Packer L, Witt EH, Tritschler HJ. Alpha-lipoic acid as a biological antioxidant. Free Radic Biol Med. 1995 Aug;19(2):227-50. Review.

Pani G, Colavitti R, Bedogni B, Fusco S, Ferraro D, Borrello S, Galeotti T. Mitochondrial superoxide dismutase: a promising target for new anticancer therapies. Curr Med Chem. 2004 May;11(10):1299-308.

Perricone NV. Topical 5% alpha lipoic acid cream in the treatment of cutaneous rhytids. Aesthetic Surgery Journal. May/June 2000;20(3):218-22.

Perricone N, Nagy K, Horvath F, Dajko G, Uray I, Zs.Nagy I. Alpha lipoic acid (ALA) protects proteins against the hydroxyl free radical-induced alterations: rationale for its geriatric application. Arch Gerontol Geriatr. 1999 Jul-Aug;29(1):45-56.

Phillips SJ. Physiology of wound healing and surgical wound care. ASAIO J. 2000 Nov-Dec;46(6):S2-S5. Review.

Pobezhimova TP, Voinikov VK. Biochemical and physiological aspects of ubiquinone function. Membr Cell Biol. 2000;13(5):595-602. Review.

Podda M, Rallis M, Traber MG, Packer L, Maibach HI. Kinetic study of cutaneous and subcutaneous distribution following topical application of [7,8-14C]rac-alpha-lipoic acid onto hairless mice. Biochem Pharmacol. 1996 Aug 23;52(4):627-33.

Podda M, Tritschler HJ, Ulrich H, Packer L. Alpha-lipoic acid supplementation prevents symptoms of vitamin E deficiency. Biochem Biophys Res Commun. 1994 Oct 14;204(1):98-104.

Podda M, Zollner TM, Grundmann-Kollmann M, Thiele JJ, Packer L, Kaufmann R. Activity of alpha-lipoic acid in the protection against oxidative stress in skin. Curr Probl Dermatol. 2001;29:43-51.

Preedy VR, Patel VB, Reilly ME, Richardson PJ, Falkous G, Mantle D. Oxidants, antioxidants and alcohol: implications for skeletal and cardiac muscle. Front Biosci. 1999 Aug 1;4:e58-e66.

Price DL, Rhett PM, Thorpe SR, Baynes JW. Chelating activity of advanced glycation end-product inhibitors. J Biol Chem. 2001 Dec 28;276(52):48967-72. Epub October 24, 2001.

Quinn PJ, Boldyrev AA, Formazuyk VE. Carnosine: its properties, functions and potential therapeutic applications. Mol Aspects Med. 1992;13(5):379-444.

Reber F, Geffarth R, Kasper M, Reichenbach A, Schleicher ED, Siegner A, Funk RH. Graded sensitiveness of the various retinal neuron populations on the glyoxal-mediated formation of advanced glycation end products and ways of protection. Graefes Arch Clin Exp Ophthalmol. 2003 Mar;241(3):213-25. Epub February 7, 2003.

Reynolds TM. The future of nutrition and wound healing. J Tissue Viability. 2001 Jan;11(1):5-13. Review.

Riserus U, Berglund L, Vessby B. Conjugated linoleic acid (CLA) reduced abdominal adipose tissue in obese middle-aged men with signs of the metabolic syndrome: a randomised controlled trial. Int J Obes Relat Metab Disord. 2001 Aug;25(8):1129-35.

Roberts PR, Zaloga GP. Cardiovascular effects of carnosine. Biochemistry (Mosc). 2000 Jul;65(7):856-61.

Rosenfeldt F, Hilton D, Pepe S, Krum H. Systematic review of effect of coenzyme Q10 in physical exercise, hypertension and heart failure. Biofactors. 2003;18(1-4):91-100. Review.

Roy S, Sen CK, Tritschler HJ, Packer L. Modulation of cellular reducing equivalent homeostasis by alpha-lipoic acid. Mechanisms and implications for diabetes and ischemic injury. Biochem Pharmacol. 1997 Feb 7;53(3):393-9.

Saliou C, Kitazawa M, McLaughlin L, Yang JP, Lodge JK, Tetsuka T, Iwasaki K, Cillard J, Okamoto T, Packer L. Antioxidants modulate acute solar ultraviolet radiation-induced NF-kappa-B activation in a human keratinocyte cell line. Free Radic Biol Med. 1999 Jan;26(1-2):174-83.

Sen CK, Packer L. Antioxidant and redox regulation of gene transcription. FASEB J. 1996;10:709-20.

Serbinova E, Kagan V, Han D, Packer L. Free radical recycling and intramembrane mobility in the antioxidant properties of alpha-tocopherol and alpha-tocotrienol. Free Radic Biol Med. 1991;10(5):263-75.

Serbinova EA, Packer L. Antioxidant properties of alpha-tocopherol and alpha-tocotrienol. Methods Enzymol. 1994;234:354-66.

Shewmake KB, Talbert GE, Bowser-Wallace BH, Caldwell FT Jr, Cone JB. Alterations in plasma copper, zinc, and ceruloplasmin levels in patients with thermal trauma. J Burn Care Rehabil. 1988 Jan-Feb;9(1):13-7.

Simeonov S, Pavlova M, Mitkov M, Mincheva L, Troev D. Therapeutic efficacy of "Milgamma" in patients with painful diabetic neuropathy. Folia Med (Plovdiv).

1997;39(4):5-10.

Stracke H, Lindemann A, Federlin K. A benfotiamine-vitamin B combination in treatment of diabetic polyneuropathy. Exp Clin Endocrinol Diabetes. 1996;104(4):311-6.

Stuerenburg HJ. The roles of carnosine in aging of skeletal muscle and in neuromuscular diseases. Biochemistry (Mosc). 2000 Jul;65(7):862-5.

Suzuki YJ, Aggarwal BB, Packer L. Alpha-lipoic acid is a potent inhibitor of NF-kappa B activation in human T cells. Biochem Biophys Res Commun. 1992 Dec 30;189(3):1709-15.

Suzuki YJ, Mizuno M, Tritschler HJ, Packer L. Redox regulation of NF-kappa B DNA binding activity by dihydrolipoate. Biochem Mol Biol Int. 1995 Jun;36(2):241-6.

Suzuki YJ, Tsuchiya M, Packer L. Lipoate prevents glucose-induced protein modifications. Free Radic Res Commun. 1992;17(3):211-7.

Swearengin TA, Fitzgerald C, Seidler NW. Carnosine prevents glyceraldehyde 3-phosphate-mediated inhibition of aspartate aminotransferase. Arch Toxicol. 1999 Aug;73(6):307-9.

Thiele JJ, Traber MG, Packer L. Depletion of human stratum corneum vitamin E: an early and sensitive in vivo marker of UV induced photo-oxidation. J Invest Dermatol. 1998 May;110(5):756-61.

Traber MG, Rallis M, Podda M, Weber C, Maibach HI, Packer L. Penetration and distribution of alpha-tocopherol, alpha- or gamma-tocotrienols applied individually onto murine skin. Lipids. 1998 Jan;33(1):87-91.

Traber, MG, et al. Diet derived topically applied tocotrienols accumulate in skin and protect the tissue against UV light-induced oxidative stress. Asia Pac J Clin Nutr. 1997;6:63-7.

Vaxman F, Olender S, Lambert A, Nisand G, Grenier JF. Can the wound healing process be improved by vitamin supplementation? Experimental study on humans. Eur Surg Res. 1996 Jul-Aug;28(4):306-14.

Wahle KW, Heys SD. Cell signal mechanisms, conjugated linoleic acids (CLAs) and anti-tumorigenesis. Prostaglandins Leukot Essent Fatty Acids. 2002 Aug-Sep;67(2-3):183-6. Review.

Weimann BI, Hermann D. Studies on wound healing: effects of calcium D-pantothenate on the migration, proliferation and protein synthesis of human dermal fibroblasts in culture. Int J Vitam Nutr Res. 1999 Mar;69(2):113-9.

Williams L. Assessing patients' nutritional needs in the wound-healing process. J Wound Care. 2002 Jun;11(6):225-8. Review.

Winkler G, Pal B, Nagybeganyi E, Ory I, Porochnavec M, Kempler P. Effectiveness of different benfotiamine dosage regimens in the treatment of painful diabetic neuropathy. Arzneimittelforschung. 1999 Mar;49(3):220-4.

Yoshida Y, Niki E, Noguchi N. Comparative study on the action of tocopherols and tocotrienols as antioxidant: chemical and physical effects. Chem Phys Lipids. 2003 Mar;123(1):63-75.

Zaloga GP, Roberts PR, Black KW, Lin M, Zapata-Sudo G, Sudo RT, Nelson TE. Carnosine is a novel peptide modulator of intracellular calcium and contractility in cardiac cells. Am J Physiol. 1997 Jan;272(1 Pt 2):H462-H468.

Ziegler D, Reljanovic M, Mehnert H, Gries FA. Alpha-lipoic acid in the treatment of diabetic polyneuropathy in Germany: current evidence from clinical trials. Exp Clin Endocrinol Diabetes. 1999;107(7):421-30. Review.

Chapter 8

Arion VY, Zimina IV, Lopuchin YM. Contemporary views on the nature and clinical application of thymus preparations. Russ J Immunol. 1997 Dec;2(3-4):157-66.

Association of Early Childhood Educators, Ontario, Canada. The importance of touch for children. Posted August 1997 at http://collections.ic.gc.ca/child/docs/00000949.htm.

Balasubramaniam A. Clinical potentials of neuropeptide Y family of hormones. Am J Surg. 2002 Apr;183(4):430-4. Review.

Ben-Efraim S, Keisari Y, Ophir R, Pecht M, Trainin N, Burstein Y. Immunopotentiating and immunotherapeutic effects of thymic hormones and factors with special emphasis on thymic humoral factor THF-gamma2. Crit Rev Immunol. 1999;19(4):261-84. Review.

Berczi I, Chalmers IM, Nagy E, Warrington RJ. The immune effects of neuropeptides. Baillieres Clin Rheumatol. 1996 May;10(2):227-57. Review.

Bierhaus A, Chevion S, Chevion M, Hofmann M, Quehenberger P, Illmer T, Luther T, Berentshtein E, Tritschler H, Muller M, Wahl P, Ziegler R, Nawroth PP. Advanced glycation end product-induced activation of NF-kappaB is suppressed by alpha-lipoic acid in cultured endothelial cells. Diabetes. 1997 Sep;46(9):1481-90.

Black PH. Stress and the inflammatory response: a review of neurogenic inflammation. Brain Behav Immun. 2002 Dec;16(6):622-53. Review.

Bodey B. Thymic hormones in cancer diagnostics and treatment. Expert Opin Biol Ther. 2001 Jan;1(1):93-107. Review.

Bodey B, Bodey B Jr, Siegel SE, Kaiser HE. Review of thymic hormones in cancer diagnosis and treatment. Int J Immunopharmacol. 2000 Apr;22(4):261-73. Review.

Cakatay U, Telci A, Kayali R, Sivas A, Akcay T. Effect of alpha-lipoic acid supplementation on oxidative protein damage in the streptozotocin-diabetic rat. Res Exp Med (Berl). 2000 Feb;199(4):243-51.

Datar P, Srivastava S, Coutinho E, Govil G. Substance P: structure, function, and therapeutics. Curr Top Med Chem. 2004;4(1):75-103. Review.

Davis TP, Konings PN. Peptidases in the CNS: formation of biologically active, receptor-specific peptide fragments. Crit Rev Neurobiol. 1993;7(3-4):163-74. Review.

Evans JL, Goldfine ID. Alpha-lipoic acid: a multifunctional antioxidant that improves insulin sensitivity in patients with type 2 diabetes. Diabetes Technol Ther. 2000 Autumn;2(3):401-13. Review.

Friedman MJ. What might the psychobiology of posttraumatic stress disorder teach us about future approaches to pharmacotherapy? J Clin Psychiatry. 2000;61 Suppl 7:44-51. Review.

Frucht-Pery J, Feldman ST, Brown SI. The use of capsaicin in herpes zoster ophthalmicus neuralgia. Acta Ophthalmol Scand. 1997 Jun;75(3):311-3.

Fuchs J, Milbradt R. Antioxidant inhibition of skin inflammation induced by reactive oxidants: evaluation of the redox couple dihydrolipoate/lipoate. Skin Pharmacol. 1994;7(5):278-84.

Galli L, de Martino M, Azzari C, Bernardini R, Cozza G, de Marco A, Lucarini D, Sabatini C, Vierucci A. [Preventive effect of thymomodulin in recurrent respiratory infections in children.] Pediatr Med Chir. 1990 May-Jun;12(3):229-32. Italian.

Gambert SR, Garthwaite TL, Pontzer CH, Cook EE, Tristani FE, Duthie EH, Martinson DR, Hagen TC, McCarty DJ. Running elevates plasma beta-endorphin immunoreactivity and ACTH in untrained human subjects. Proc Soc Exp Biol Med. 1981 Oct;168(1):1-4.

Geenen V, Kecha O, Brilot F, Hansenne I, Renard C, Martens H. Thymic T-cell tolerance of neuroendocrine functions: physiology and pathophysiology. Cell Mol Biol (Noisy-le-grand). 2001 Feb;47(1):179-88. Review.

Gianoulakis C. Implications of endogenous opioids and dopamine in alcoholism: human and basic science studies. Alcohol Alcohol Suppl. 1996 Mar;1:33-42. Review.

Girolomoni G, Giannetti A. [Neuropeptides and the skin: morphological, functional and physiopathological aspects.] G Ital Dermatol Venereol. 1989 Apr;124(4):121-40. Review. Italian.

Goldstein AL, Badamchian M. Thymosins: chemistry and biological properties in health and disease. Expert Opin Biol Ther. 2004 Apr;4(4):559-73.

Goldstein AL, Schulof RS, Naylor PH, Hall NR. Thymosins and anti-thymosins: properties and clinical applications. Med Oncol Tumor Pharmacother. 1986;3(3-4):211-21. Review.

Goya RG, Console GM, Herenu CB, Brown OA, Rimoldi OJ. Thymus and aging: potential of gene therapy for restoration of endocrine thymic function in thymus-deficient animal models. Gerontology. 2002 Sep-Oct;48(5):325-8.

Gutzwiller JP, Degen L, Matzinger D, Prestin S, Beglinger C. Interaction between GLP-1 and CCK33 in inhibiting food intake and appetite in men. Am J Physiol Regul Integr Comp Physiol. 2004 Apr 22.

Hagen TM, Liu J, Lykkesfeldt J, Wehr CM, Ingersoll RT, Vinarsky V, Bartholomew JC, Ames BN. Feeding acetyl-L-carnitine and lipoic acid to old rats significantly improves metabolic function while decreasing oxidative stress. Proc Natl Acad Sci USA. 2002 Feb 19;99(4):1870-5. Erratum in: Proc Natl Acad Sci USA. 2002 May 14;99(10):7184.

Han D, Handelman G, Marcocci L, Sen CK, Roy S, Kobuchi H, Tritschler HJ, Flohe L, Packer L. Lipoic acid increases de novo synthesis of cellular glutathione by improving cystine utilization. Biofactors. 1997;6(3):321-38.

Hill AJ, Peikin SR, Ryan CA, Blundell JE. Oral administration of proteinase inhibitor II from potatoes reduces energy intake in man. Physiol Behav. 1990 Aug;48(2):241-6.

Holmes A, Heilig M, Rupniak NM, Steckler T, Griebel G. Neuropeptide systems as novel therapeutic targets for depression and anxiety disorders. Trends Pharmacol Sci. 2003 Nov;24(11):580-8.

Hughes J, Kosterlitz HW, Smith TW. The distribution of methionine-enkephalin and leucine-enkephalin in the brain and peripheral tissues. 1977. Br J Pharmacol. 1997 eb;120 (Suppl 4):428-36, discussion 426-7.

arvikallio A, Harvima IT, Naukkarinen A. Mast cells, nerves and neuropeptides in atopic dermatitis and nummular eczema. Arch Dermatol Res. 2003 Apr;295(1):2-7. Epub January 31, 2003.

essop DS, Harbuz MS, Lightman SL. CRH in chronic inflammatory stress. Peptides. 2001 May;22(5):803-7. Review.

Kagan VE, Shvedova A, Serbinova E, Khan S, Swanson C, Powell R, Packer L. Dihydrolipoic acid—a universal antioxidant both in the membrane and in the aqueous phase. Reduction of peroxyl, ascorbyl and chromanoxyl radicals. Biochem Pharmacol. 1992 Oct 20;44(8):1637-49.

Kastin AJ, Zadina JE, Olson RD, Banks WA. The history of neuropeptide research: version 5.a. Ann NY Acad Sci. 1996 Mar 22;780:1-18. Review.

Katsuno M, Aihara M, Kojima M, Osuna H, Hosoi J, Nakamura M, Toyoda M, Matsuda H, Ikezawa Z. Neuropeptide concentrations in the skin of a murine (NC/Nga mice) model of atopic dermatitis. J Dermatol Sci. 2003 Oct;33(1):55-65.

Khavinson VKh. Peptides and ageing. Neuroendocrinol Lett. 2002;23 Suppl 3:11-144. Review.

Khavinson VKh, Morozov VG. Peptides of pineal gland and thymus prolong human life. Neuroendocrinol Lett. 2003 Jun-Aug;24(3-4):233-40.

Kocak G, Aktan F, Canbolat O, Ozogul C, Elbeg S, Yildizoglu-Ari N, Karasu C. Alpha-lipoic acid treatment ameliorates metabolic parameters, blood pressure, vascular reactivity and morphology of vessels already damaged by streptozotocin-diabetes. Diabetes Nutr Metab. 2000 Dec;13(6):308-18.

Komarcevic A. [The modern approach to wound treatment.] Med Pregl. 2000 Jul-Aug;53(7-8):363-8. Review. Croatian.

Kosterlitz HW, Corbett AD, Paterson SJ. Opioid receptors and ligands. NIDA Res Monogr. 1989;95:159-66. Review.

Kouttab NM, Prada M, Cazzola P. Thymomodulin: biological properties and clinical applications. Med Oncol Tumor Pharmacother. 1989;6(1):5-9. Review.

Kramer MS, Winokur A, Kelsey J, Preskorn SH, Rothschild AJ, Snavely D, Ghosh K, Ball WA, Reines SA, Munjack D, Apter JT, Cunningham L, Kling M, Bari M, Getson A, Lee Y. Demonstration of the efficacy and safety of a novel Substance P (NK1) receptor antagonist in major depression. Neuropsychopharmacology. 2004 Feb;29(2):385-92.

Kunt T, et al. Alpha-lipoic acid reduces expression of vascular cell adhesion molecule-1 and endothelial adhesion of human monocytes after stimulation with advanced glycation end products. Clin Sci (Lond). 1999 Jan;96(1):75-82.

Li L, Zhou JH, Xing ST, Chen ZR. [Effect of thymic factor D on lipid peroxide, glutathione, and membrane fluidity in liver of aged rats.] Zhongguo Yao Li Xue Bao. 1993 Jul;14(4):382-4. Chinese.

Linetsky M, James HL, Ortwerth BJ. Spontaneous generation of superoxide anion by human lens proteins and by calf lens proteins ascorbylated in vitro. Exp Eye Res. 1999 Aug;69(2):239-48.

Low TL, Goldstein AL. Thymosins: structure, function and therapeutic applications.

Thymus. 1984;6(1-2):27-42. Review.

Maiorano V, Chianese R, Fumarulo R, Costantino E, Contini M, Carnimeo R, Cazzola P. Thymomodulin increases the depressed production of superoxide anion by alveolar macrophages in patients with chronic bronchitis. Int J Tissue React. 1989;11(1):21-5.

Martin-Du-Pan RC. [Thymic hormones. Neuroendocrine interactions and clinical use in congenital and acquired immune deficiencies.] Ann Endocrinol (Paris) 1984;45(6):355-68. Review. French.

Melhem MF, Craven PA, DeRubertis FR. Effects of dietary supplementation of alpha-lipoic acid on early glomerular injury in diabetes mellitus. J Am Soc Nephrol. 2001 Jan;12(1):124-33.

Melhem MF, Craven PA, Liachenko J, DeRubertis FR. Alpha-lipoic acid attenuates hyperglycemia and prevents glomerular mesangial matrix expansion in diabetes. J Am Soc Nephrol. 2002 Jan;13(1):108-16.

Meyer M, Pahl HL, Baeuerle PA. Regulation of the transcription factors NF-kappa B and AP-1 by redox changes. Chem Biol Interact. 1994 Jun;91(2-3):91-100.

Meyer M, Schreck R, Baeuerle PA. H2O2 and antioxidants have opposite effects on activation of NF-kappa B and AP-1 in intact cells: AP-1 as secondary antioxidant-responsive factor. EMBO J. 1993 May;12(5):2005-15.

Midaoui AE, Elimadi A, Wu L, Haddad PS, de Champlain J. Lipoic acid prevents hypertension, hyperglycemia, and the increase in heart mitochondrial superoxide production. Am J Hypertens. 2003 Mar;16(3):173-9.

Misery L. Skin, immunity and the nervous system. Br J Dermatol. 1997 Dec;137(6):843-50. Review.

Morgan CA 3rd, Wang S, Southwick SM, Rasmusson A, Hazlett G, Hauger RL, Charney DS. Plasma Neuropeptide-Y concentrations in humans exposed to military survival training. Biol Psychiatry. 2000 May 15;47(10):902-9.

Obrenovich ME, Monnier VM. Vitamin B1 blocks damage caused by hyperglycemia. Sci Aging Knowledge Environ. 2003 Mar 12;2003(10):PE6.

Ookawara T, Kawamura N, Kitagawa Y, Taniguchi N. Site-specific and random fragmentation of Cu,Zn-superoxide dismutase by glycation reaction. Implication of reactive oxygen species. J Biol Chem. 1992 Sep 15;267(26):18505-10.

Pacher P, Kecskemeti V. Trends in the development of new antidepressants. Is there a light at the end of the tunnel? Curr Med Chem. 2004 Apr;11(7):925-43.

Pacher P, Kohegyi E, Kecskemeti V, Furst S. Current trends in the development of new antidepressants. Curr Med Chem. 2001 Feb;8(2):89-100. Review.

Packer L, Kraemer K, Rimbach G. Molecular aspects of lipoic acid in the prevention of diabetes complications. Nutrition. 2001 Oct;17(10):888-95. Review.

Packer L, Roy S, Sen CK. A-lipoic acid: a metabolic antioxidant and potential redox modulator of transcription. Adv Pharmacol. 1996;38:79-101.

Packer L, Witt EH, Tritschler HJ. Alpha-lipoic acid as a biological antioxidant. Free Radic Biol Med. 1995 Aug;19(2):227-50. Review.

Paez X, Hernandez L, Baptista T. [Advances in the molecular treatment of depression.] Rev Neurol. 2003 Sep 1-15;37(5):459-70. Review. Spanish.

Pani G, Colavitti R, Bedogni B, Fusco S, Ferraro D, Borrello S, Galeotti T. Mitochonrial superoxide dismutase: a promising target for new anticancer therapies. Curr Med Chem. 2004 May;11(10):1299-308.

arker J. Do It Now Foundation. http://www.doitnow.org/.

erricone NV. Topical 5% alpha lipoic acid cream in the treatment of cutaneous rhytids. esthetic Surg J. 2000 May-June; 20(3):218-22.

'erricone N, Nagy K, Horvath F, Dajko G, Uray I, Zs.Nagy I. Alpha lipoic acid (ALA) rotects proteins against the hydroxyl free radical-induced alterations: rationale for its eriatric application. Arch Gerontol Geriatr. 1999 Jul-Aug;29(1):45-56.

'ert CB, Pasternak G, Snyder SH. Opiate agonists and antagonists discriminated by eceptor binding in brain. Science. 1973 Dec 28;182(119):1359-61.

'odda M, Rallis M, Traber MG, Packer L, Maibach HI. Kinetic study of cutaneous and ubcutaneous distribution following topical application of [7,8-14C]rac-alpha-lipoic cid onto hairless mice. Biochem Pharmacol. 1996 Aug 23;52(4):627-33.

'odda M, Tritschler HJ, Ulrich H, Packer L. Alpha-lipoic acid supplementation prevents ymptoms of vitamin E deficiency. Biochem Biophys Res Commun. 1994 Oct 4;204(1):98-104.

'odda M, Zollner TM, Grundmann-Kollmann M, Thiele JJ, Packer L, Kaufmann R. Activity of alpha-lipoic acid in the protection against oxidative stress in skin. Curr Probl Dermatol. 2001;29:43-51.

Rains C, Bryson HM. Topical capsaicin. A review of its pharmacological properties and herapeutic potential in post-herpetic neuralgia, diabetic neuropathy and osteoarthritis. Drugs Aging. 1995 Oct;7(4):317-28. Review.

Rasmusson AM, Hauger RL, Morgan CA, Bremner JD, Charney DS, Southwick SM. Low baseline and yohimbine-stimulated plasma Neuropeptide Y (NPY) levels in ombat-related PTSD. Biol Psychiatry. 2000 Mar 15;47(6):526-39.

Reber F, Geffarth R, Kasper M, Reichenbach A, Schleicher ED, Siegner A, Funk RH. Graded sensitiveness of the various retinal neuron populations on the glyoxal-mediated ormation of advanced glycation end products and ways of protection. Graefes Arch Clin Exp Ophthalmol. 2003 Mar;241(3):213-25. Epub February 7, 2003.

Roy S, Sen CK, Tritschler HJ, Packer L. Modulation of cellular reducing equivalent homeostasis by alpha-lipoic acid. Mechanisms and implications for diabetes and schemic injury. Biochem Pharmacol. 1997 Feb 7;53(3):393-9.

Saliou C, Kitazawa M, McLaughlin L, Yang JP, Lodge JK, Tetsuka T, Iwasaki K, Cillard J, Okamoto T, Packer L. Antioxidants modulate acute solar ultraviolet radiation-induced NF-kappa-B activation in a human keratinocyte cell line. Free Radic Biol Med. 1999 Jan;26(1-2):174-83.

Schulof RS. Thymic peptide hormones: basic properties and clinical applications in cancer. Crit Rev Oncol Hematol. 1985;3(4):309-76. Review.

Sen CK, Packer L. Antioxidant and redox regulation of gene transcription. FASEB J. 1996;10:709-20.

Silva AP, Cavadas C, Grouzmann E. Neuropeptide Y and its receptors as potential therapeutic drug targets. Clin Chim Acta. 2002 Dec;326(1-2):3-25. Review.

Suzuki YJ, Aggarwal BB, Packer L. Alpha-lipoic acid is a potent inhibitor of NF-kappa

B activation in human T cells. Biochem Biophys Res Commun. 1992 Dec 30;189(3):1709-15.

Suzuki YJ, Mizuno M, Tritschler HJ, Packer L. Redox regulation of NF-kappa B DNA binding activity by dihydrolipoate. Biochem Mol Biol Int. 1995 Jun;36(2):241-6.

Suzuki YJ, Tsuchiya M, Packer L. Lipoate prevents glucose-induced protein modifications. Free Radic Res Commun. 1992;17(3):211-7.

Tada H, Nakashima A, Awaya A, Fujisaki A, Inoue K, Kawamura K, Itoh K, Masuda H, Suzuki T. Effects of thymic hormone on reactive oxygen species-scavengers and renal function in tacrolimus-induced nephrotoxicity. Life Sci. 2002 Jan 25;70(10):1213-23.

Toyoda M, Morohashi M. New aspects in acne inflammation. Dermatology 2003;206(1):17-23. Review.

Toyoda M, Nakamura M, Makino T, Hino T, Kagoura M, Morohashi M. Nerve growth factor and Substance P are useful plasma markers of disease activity in atopic dermatitis. Br J Dermatol. 2002 Jul;147(1):71-9.

Toyoda M, Nakamura M, Morohashi M. Neuropeptides and sebaceous glands. Eur J Dermatol. 2002 Sep-Oct;12(5):422-7. Review.

Ziegler D, Reljanovic M, Mehnert H, Gries FA. Alpha-lipoic acid in the treatment of diabetic polyneuropathy in Germany: current evidence from clinical trials. Exp Clin Endocrinol Diabetes. 1999;107(7):421-30. Review.

Index